# Remaking Chronic Care in the Age of Health Care Reform

# Remaking Chronic Care in the Age of Health Care Reform

## Changes for Lower Cost, Higher Quality Treatment

Arnold Birenbaum

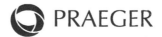 PRAEGER

AN IMPRINT OF ABC-CLIO, LLC
Santa Barbara, California • Denver, Colorado • Oxford, England

**Library of Congress Cataloging-in-Publication Data**

Birenbaum, Arnold.
    Remaking chronic care in the age of health care reform : changes for lower cost, higher quality treatment / Arnold Birenbaum.
        p. ; cm.
    Includes bibliographical references and index.
    ISBN 978–0–313–39888–9 (hard copy : alk. paper) — ISBN 978–0–313–39889–6 (ebook)
1. Long-term care of the sick—United States. 2. Health care reform—United States. 3. United States. Patient Protection and Affordable Care Act. I. Title.
[DNLM: 1. United States. Patient Protection and Affordable Care Act. 2. Long-Term Care—economics—United States. 3. Chronic Disease—economics—United States. 4. Health Care Reform—United States. 5. Quality of Health Care—United States. WX 162]
RA997.B57    2011
362.1068′1—dc23                    2011017324

ISBN: 978–0–313–39888–9
EISBN: 978–0–313–39889–6

15  14  13  12  11      1  2  3  4  5

This book is also available on the World Wide Web as an eBook.
Visit www.abc-clio.com for details.

Praeger
An Imprint of ABC-CLIO, LLC

ABC-CLIO, LLC
130 Cremona Drive, P.O. Box 1911
Santa Barbara, California 93116-1911

This book is printed on acid-free paper ∞

Manufactured in the United States of America

*For Naomi and Rebecca,
the granddaughters from California*

# Contents

# Preface

Chronic illness and its care in the United States is a subject that is of major concern in an aging society. It is often the case that both public and private insurance, as well as out-of-pocket expenditures, as utilized, do not always realize improved quality of life, prevent declines, or ward off death. Failure to receive appropriate chronic care is a major social problem since individuals are left without the opportunity to use their skills and talents to attain security, recognition, and self-regard.

In fact, a society could be judged ethically according to how well citizens are able to achieve a capacity to use their freedoms to choose to follow their dreams and do things that are meaningful to them, according to the Nobel laureate economist Amartya Sen (2010). To some of us old-timers, this statement is much in the spirit of Franklin Delano Roosevelt's Four Freedoms. To Samuel Freeman (2010), in reviewing Sen's *The Idea of Justice*, this freedom, in summary, sits on a foundation of social support.

> Important capabilities include have adequate nutrition; health and longevity; personal safety and freedom from fear; physical mobility, literacy and numeracy; and being able to appear in public without shame. (p. 58)

Chronic illness often calls into question the capacity of a society to distribute fairly these supports. The absence of this capacity has brought forth impressive advocates, both among the chronically ill and within the healing professions. The problems of chronic care have generated some exciting opportunities to remake it, even in a society where many of its citizens have misunderstood and therefore not fully embraced the systems-change benefits of recent health care reform legislation. Despite a movement that propels forward changes in the financial and delivery system of chronic care, writing about its remaking is a sometimes elusive task. It is far less concrete a subject and therefore a more challenging task than attempting to write about the impact of managed care on the independence and dominance of medicine—a subject of great interest in the early part of this century—one that I wrote about (Birenbaum, 2002).

The narrative of the remaking of chronic care requires putting together various strands of advocacy and reform, largely lead by primary care avatars within the medical profession, often in the name of patients and large employers in the United States who find the cost of health care benefits for current workers and the retired as unsustainable. Despair has not been an option and there have been pockets of nonprofit enterprise and government entrepreneurship to turn things around. From different parts of the country, financing and delivery experiments were attempted in creating patient-centered medical homes, accountable care organizations, and bundled payment formulas, a three-legged stool that can gain public support for improvements in the quality of care as well as cost reductions. Yet these subjects do not exactly leave the U.S. public in thrall.

Buttressing these efforts to redesign care systems, generally to deal with the ineffectiveness and inefficiencies in furnishing chronic care, are elegant studies of how there are some localities that deliver quality care to everyone at reasonable cost. The research techniques for identifying these communities have been quietly cultivated for more than 25 years. The comparative research of the Dartmouth Atlas of Health Care, under the direction of John Wennberg and Elliott Fisher, has spotlighted some regions where medical expenditures are low and Medicare patients live long lives, as in the celebrated story of Grand Junction, Colorado (Bodenheimer and West, 2010). The availability of comparative performance and its measurement in the field of healthcare delivery has made it possible to say that sometimes less care is more or at least of better value for patients. Grand Junction was not only made available to the reading public in major articles in national magazines but also visited by President Barack Obama in his effort to rally support for the somewhat arcane contents of the Patient Protection and Affordable Care Act (PPACA) on its way to becoming law.

As a result of these challenging studies, as well as the media-covered visit from the Commander in Chief during the run-up to the passage of health reform legislation in the spring of 2010, a great deal of attention has been paid recently to this subject in the health care delivery and financing as well as in the advocacy literature. The status quo is largely unacceptable and unsustainable and this current state speaks to the critical need for change. Fortunately, health care planners are not starting from scratch; there are some remedies in the pipeline but major changes in the health delivery and financing system can take 15 years to implement.

There is some momentum building both related to covering the uninsured and making for better results through improvements in chronic care. Congress and the President of the United States weighed in with transformative legislation in 2010 that attempts to deal with the fundamental financial insecurities for individuals in the face of chronic illness, provides support for research to find out what works, and underwrites large-scale efforts to introduce better ways of caring for this part of the population. In so doing, the goal of these initiatives is to reverse the out-of-control course of our health care system's expenditures, the decline in quality, and the need for a better way to help people manage with conditions that are of lifelong duration and that interfere with the quality of life.

For Americans with chronic health conditions—hypertension, heart disease, diabetes, or arthritis, to name but a few of the diseases for which there are no cures—there may be little help available that can be applied proactively. In other words, while there are many interventions for people with chronic illnesses that can be made to improve their quality of life and avoid hospital admissions, they may not get what they need when they need it. A person living with a chronic illness who shows up at the emergency department of a community or teaching hospital in an acute and deteriorating state will surely be hospitalized as a precaution. Some recently published commentaries, with the emphasis on sophisticated primary care delivered via the patient-centered medical home, suggest that we can do better, get greater valued for the money spent, and spend less on health care. According to data collected by the Center on Medicare and Medicaid Services, 10 percent of Medicare patients account for 64 percent of costs, and many of these patients are afflicted with chronic conditions. Bending the cost curve, a favorite expression among policy experts, means more money available for other vital services such as education.

The promise of quality care at lower cost requires the redesign of health services and how they are paid for. Along with the idea of the medical home there is recent advocacy among health policy analysts and system designers of the accountable care organization, a way to prevent the frequent rehospitalization of anywhere from one third to one fifth of Medicare patients within 30 days of discharge, depending on the geographic location. Many of these patients have one or more chronic diseases and need coordinated and continuous care when they undergo transition to the community. Aligning payments and incentives to providers to support coordination is a major way to create better chronic care.

Both the patient-centered medical home and accountable care organizations are supported in the Patient Protection and Affordable Care Act, now increasingly referred to in the press, recent health policy literature, and in the electronic media as the Affordable Care Act. Barely six months old as I write, there are some hopeful signs that change is coming. There are various innovations that are coming together, allowing providers and managed care plans to connect the new efforts to digitalize patient information, permitting them to use that information to both assist patients and create performance measures. In doing so, the leaders in health care reform on the ground are reinventing the health care infrastructure and provider incentives that are compatible with the new health care reform law. There is a need to furnish the full narrative to these amazing signs of progress and how we can make a comeback nationally from a deteriorated and fragmented state of contemporary health care.

This book attempts to show the current critical condition of chronic care, the compatibility of change in incentives as encouraged by the Affordable Care Act, and what we have learned about ways to fuel improvements in the locus and quality of care. *Remaking Chronic Care in the Age of Health Care Reform: Changes for Lower Cost, Higher Quality Treatment* is a scholarly work based on the most recent demographic studies of *which* sectors of the U.S. population contribute disproportionately to our current chronic care needs, the possible explanations for this phenomenon, and the extensive research on how the health care system attempts to respond or stumbles when it comes to chronic illness.

What is fascinating and encouraging about these attempts at reform is that they are often coming from within the profession of medicine and from hospitals and health care systems that want to do the right thing. These innovations do not involve, as some on the Right might have it, the federal government demanding that one size fits all. In fact, for-profit insurers were guiltier than the U.S. Department of

Health and Human Service officials for imposing limits on how care was to be delivered.

There were always some physicians who led the charge for creating value in health care, usually because they had unusual work environments where patients were covered via capitation payment systems. Following the push-back in the 1990s from hospitals and physicians against the rigidities of insurance company directed managed care plans, some reformist elements started to build new ways of assisting physicians who were seriously interested in improving patient care. These programs grew in few places but the innovators persisted in making them viable as professional organizations. The origins of the innovations in service delivery and evidence for their success are initially identified in the chronic care model, as introduced in Seattle, Washington, at the celebrated Group Health Cooperative.

Still, it must be noted that one size does not fit all people. Not all populations are easily adaptable to the chronic care model. Special attention is paid in this volume to the problems of access and affordability to chronic care by people with disabilities and multiple chronic conditions. To view chronic care from a consumer's perspective, I include, whenever possible, patient satisfaction data and consumer quotations elicited from individuals with regard to experiences with the patient-centered medical home and accountable care organizations.

Issues related to financing—from an individual, commercial, and social insurance perspective—are addressed in later chapters. Shortfalls in capacity to produce systems change are noted. As the Affordable Care Act attempts to overcome some of the problems related to how innovative health care services for people with chronic illnesses will be paid for, the strong reliance on primary care in public insurance programs such as Medicare and Medicaid may be called into question by the limited capacity of the medical and advanced practice nursing educational and training systems to produce primary care providers in sufficient numbers to redesign health care delivery in what has become the age of chronic care. Finally, all of the ways in which the Affordable Care Act affects chronic care will be discussed in the concluding chapter.

I have attempted to keep the information I introduce in the chapters fresh, and scholarly journals, newspapers, and magazines have helped enormously with an information blizzard that is beyond belief. This book project has been in development since June 2009 and the progress I made in 2009 and 2010 was possible because I had superb support. These efforts have to be acknowledged. I was greatly assisted by the excellent organizational skills of Midori Euhara, at that time an unpaid intern and an undergraduate at Stanford University, interested in learning more about the health care system of the United States and the broad issues related to reform. Having collected a great number of journal articles, newspaper accounts, and policy briefs, I was blessed by her presence for most of the summer of 2009 and her ability to link up the various sources of information to the general chapter outlines. I know for certain that Midori learned a great deal about health care reform and will use her "big picture" intellect to add value to whatever she does professionally.

New articles continued to appear during 2009 and 2010 since the subject of remaking chronic care, accountable care organizations, patient-centered medical homes, and bundled payment received a great deal of attention in the scholarly literature as well as in weekly magazines and the daily newspapers. I was assisted by Phyllis Angelico in keeping these references organized as well as in the creation of the tables found in the book. In addition, she was an excellent source of homemade pastries, especially around Christmas 2010.

What I was writing during these months was subject to some content review. An earlier draft of *Remaking Chronic Care* was read carefully by Susan Yuan, a colleague in the intellectual and developmental disability field and a parent of a young adult with complex health problems as well as a disability. Susan was a careful reader of the manuscript and made important observations about what could be improved. More specifically, her guidance was invaluable in showing me some of the dilemmas faced by people with disabilities in an emotionally distant and cold health care system.

My dear old friend and fellow sociologist Martin Wenglinsky was also a dedicated reader of the manuscript and offered a great deal of useful criticism. I have learned from his always cogent and sometimes profound commentaries. He has urged me to see this enterprise as a way of understanding the complexities of institution building when there are so many barriers to achieving better quality care at lower cost. His openness to the world of ideas is an inspiration, particularly since the full story of the causes, conduct, and consequences of the remaking of chronic care cannot be told simply by summarizing empirical studies about where quality improvements make a difference and how much can be saved cost-wise in a health care system that is wasteful and dollar driven.

# Chronic Care: An Introduction

Chronic care in the United States is the arena where the personal, economic, and political in our current turbulent era often meet, albeit awkwardly. Those who deny the tensions in this kind of encounter often fail to see their own vulnerabilities and the need for human beings to be part of something larger than the lone individual. The presence of disease reminds us of this simple fact. Public insurers such as Medicare and Medicaid are being revisited by health policy analysts not only to eliminate waste but also to establish more effective delivery systems. Even insurance companies are starting to see the wisdom of making resources available to primary care physicians so that they can assist patients with multiple chronic illnesses or even a single serious condition (Abelson, 2010a, p. B1).

This is no small paradigmatic breakthrough in a land where claims for payments for care or medications are often denied in quite arbitrary ways and where unnecessary treatment takes place because of the financial stakes involved. There are good reasons to reverse some of these current practices that do not help people manage their chronic illnesses. For starters, we note that a sick person is a psychologically and socially vulnerable person. Most modern societies recognize the need to eliminate barriers to access to health care for the sick as well as helping to keep people well. Congress and the President of the United States weighed in in 2010 with far-reaching legislation that attempts to deal with the fundamental financial insecurities in the face of chronic illness, find out what works, and make large-scale efforts to introduce better ways of caring for this part of the population. In so doing, the goal of these initiatives is to reverse the out-of-control course of our health care system and help people manage with conditions that are of prolonged duration and rarely cured.

The late Susan Sontag (1978), a brilliant and compelling writer and a long-time cancer patient, captured the meaning of illness as the acquisition of new responsibilities, albeit unwanted ones.

> Illness is the night-side of life, a more onerous citizenship. Everyone who is born holds dual citizenship, in the kingdom of the well and the kingdom of the sick. Although we all prefer to use only the good passport, sooner or later each of us is obliged at least to identify ourselves as citizens of that other place. (p. 10)

The strain of managing emotionally and with regard to social relationships is evident in the new issues that must be faced in playing the sick role. People who become ill face a number of uncertainties: how they will be regarded by others, whether they will be permanently impaired, and whether they will be able to lead normal lives. Dr. Julian L. Seifter, a 61-year-old nephrologist at Brigham and Women's Hospital in Boston, is a subspecialist who treats patients with chronic kidney disease. Cleary, Dr. Seifter is working with a patient population made up of people with a severe chronic illness. What makes his work interesting is the fact that he is both a caregiver to people with chronic illnesses and a receiver of chronic care himself. He was also diagnosed with diabetes more than 30 years ago and has faced grave associated disabilities as well as the daily routine of administering insulin to himself, sticking to an austere diet, and monitoring his blood sugar levels. He has used his experience in changing his life interests and routines, and he hopes to learn how to guide his patients to give up pursuits that they love and how to establish new avocations, sometimes leading to life course changes. With limited vision related to complications of diabetes and reading made difficult, Dr. Seifter learned to try new things such as gardening as a way to find creative activities that did not put undue strain on his eyes. In an interview with Claudia Dreifus (2010), Dr. Seifter discussed his new book, coauthored with his wife Betsy Seifter, *After the Diagnosis: Transcending Chronic Illness,* and how he was able to focus on what he could still do and do well. To some degree, Dr. Seifter was able to recognize that being a nephrologist with diabetes did give him some advantages when relating to patients. Dreifus concentrated on how a life challenge can be put to good use in one's profession since Dr. Seifter does more with his patients than simply follow their renal disease. The interview did not deal with how chronic disease can alter family relationships or even how one relates to colleagues.

While chronic illnesses are not communicable, they do change people's relationship with members of their families, workmates, and the health care services that they access. Payers of health care services, whether commercial insurers or employers who help pay premiums or self-insure, and directors of public programs such as Medicare and Medicaid are acutely sensitive to the unsustainable rise in costs, largely due to financing chronic care. Payers and providers are starting, with the support of the new federal health care reform law, to strategize on how to limit costs. These partnerships are encouraging, given the limits that confine efforts at primary prevention through healthier practices in living and early identification of disease. Yet we also find that insurance plans are raising their premiums in anticipation of restrictions on rates once the new law is implemented.

Donald Berwick, a physician appointed in July 2010 by President Obama to be the Director of the Center on Medicare and Medicaid Services (CMS) and a major advocate for health care improvement, and surely in line to become our most eloquent bureaucrat, proposed in 2009 (p. w560) that patient centered care is "The experience (to the extent the informed, individual patient desires it) of transparency, individualization, recognition, respect, dignity, and choice in all matters, without exception, related to one's person, circumstances and relationships in health care " How often can we as patients claim that this is what we experienced? Is this experience possible in our large health care institutions?

There is a legislative foundation for this kind of care and the Center on Medicare and Medicaid Services has wasted no time in getting out the message that this is a new era in the United States. The new health care law, according to Secretary of Health and Human Services Kathleen Sebelius (2010a), will make available patient-centered care for Medicare-eligible individuals and will improve the quality of chronic care so that following hospitalization, at the least, a successful return home will take place and readmission will be avoided. This promise—coordinated care and greater connectivity to community services and supports—will be implemented through widespread expansion of new incentives to doctors and hospitals. Secretary Sebelius refers to the medical home as "one of the most promising models for improving the quality of care and bringing down health care costs" (qtd. in Freudenheim, 2010, p. D6). For patients who are seeing as many as seven or eight doctors, the patient-centered medical home is a necessary cure to fragmented care.

Linked up with the medical home, patient-centered care has become even more attractive, given the needs of an aging population, often involving patients with multiple chronic illnesses. And a new complex health care reform law, the Patient Protection and Affordable Care Act (PPACA), signed into law in March 2010 and with many provisions to encourage cost reduction and improvements in the quality of care, puts chronic illness on the top of the "to do better" list. It is no accident that these sections of PPACA made it into health care reform, since the patient-centered medical home not only pays off in terms of better outcomes for patients, it can also be delivered at less cost than uncoordinated care. In the melodramatic process of creating legislation that can gain enough votes in the Senate to pass, anticipated funding for the "scaling up" of the patient-centered medical home made it possible for the Congressional Budget Office to show that the bill, over time, would be budget neutral.

All of these outcomes take serious planning and time to scale-up. It appears that one of the major problems in the near term will be how to find enough primary care providers to take on all the tasks anticipated in this transformation of the U.S. health care system required to reduce dependence on hospital admissions and visits to emergency departments. Identified as a cultural movement, the patient-centered medical home has become the delivery mechanism for chronic care for veteran primary care advocates such as Eric B. Larson and Robert Reid from the Group Health Research Institute in Seattle, Washington (2010, p. 1644). In its current fractured state, U.S. health care, compared to other countries with similar standards of living, does not deliver good value considering how much is spent annually and as part of our gross domestic product.

There is strong evidence that the U.S. health care system's capacity to care for people with chronic illnesses has far to go when compared with other countries. One of our premier nonprofit health care foundations—the Commonwealth Fund—conducted telephone interviews with 7,500 adults living in Australia, Canada, France, Germany, the Netherlands, New Zealand, the United Kingdom (UK), and the United States. The focus was on people who required heavy maintenance to keep from getting sicker. Every respondent had one or more chronic health problems, including hypertension, heart disease, diabetes, arthritis, lung problems, cancer, or depression. Additionally, all had either recently been hospitalized, undergone major surgery, or had a serious episode of their illness. As reported in a *Health Affairs* Web exclusive released November 2008, the study found substantial differences in the eight countries regarding the survey participants' access to care, care coordination, and medical or medication errors.

A national system comparison, based on these experiences of chronically ill adults, indicates that health care reform in the United States must pay attention to gaps in financing and service delivery. The international comparisons are striking: Limited access due to cost barriers ranged from 7 percent in the Netherlands to 54 percent in the United States; coordination problems also showed wide variation, from 14 percent in the Netherlands to 34 percent in the United States; finally, medical, medication, or laboratory errors were reported by 17 percent of the respondents in the Netherlands versus 34 percent among Americans who participated in this international survey, conducted in 2008. Note that we are not talking about the "young invincibles," as they were designated by the media during the health care reform debate, who may get away with being uninsured in the United States, but people with medical histories that need to be attended to.

Serious chronic illness and how it is treated nation by nation reveals a great deal about what needs to be fixed in the U.S. health care system. There is also something to be learned from state-based studies when the consequences of loss of insurance coverage take place. Failure to furnish care for several major chronic conditions because insurance coverage was interrupted is also an important factor in inviting the risk of preventable hospitalizations. The results of a study of California Medicaid beneficiaries who had their coverage interrupted, reported in the *Annals of Internal Medicine* on December 16, 2008, and who suffered from heart failure, diabetes, and chronic obstructive pulmonary disease were far more likely to be hospitalized than those beneficiaries with these same chronic diseases whose coverage was maintained during the five-year study period. The authors concluded that reducing interruptions to coverage "might prevent some of the health events that trigger hospitalization and high-cost health spending" (Bindman, Chattopadhyay, and Auerback, 2008, p. 859).

Avoiding hospitalization is clearly a good thing and part of the story of how to improve chronic care. However, ambulatory care for these serious chronic illnesses, as noted in the international survey, also can be subject to disproportionately high rates of poor coordination and medical error. Any effort to maintain and extend Medicaid coverage, employer-based coverage, or market-based individual insurance during the current economic downturn needs to be supported by improvements in service delivery, particularly where outpatient care is involved. President Obama needs to be held accountable for his promises during the implementation of PPACA, where in his administration there will be movement toward coverage for all, quality care, and lower costs. As well, the enemies of PPACA need to present an alternative plan for healing our fragmented health care system that will increase the odds that people who require chronic care will get it and will be able to receive patient centered care, the kind of care that they claim will not be delivered under what they argue is a government-run health care system.

Some physicians and health delivery system planners have been aware of the critical need to fix chronic care and this concern can be documented from the policy statements made at some professional meetings, where serious attention has been paid for more than a decade as to what must be done. In November 1999, the keynote speaker at the annual meetings of the Academy on an Aging Society noted that "[c]hronic conditions are the major cause of illness, disability and death in the United States." A decade later, in the new age of health care reform, launched by the Obama administration, health delivery experts recommend that we encourage coordinated care among doctors and hospitals when it comes to addressing chronic illness.

Coordinated care can only be accomplished when there are rewards or incentives for its performance, meaning that the system has to lose the piece-work or fee-for-service payment structure that currently exists and does little to promote care coordination and is embarrassingly ineffective when it comes to cost control. In addition, hospitals that are compensated on a per diem basis for bed use might see a drop in the demand for admissions or reductions in lengths of stay if excellent community-based chronic care was available. The health care system will be sharply redesigned if this transformation to comprehensive and continuous chronic care comes forth in a robust way.

The effort to reform the health care system, driven by PPACA, reveals a great concern on the part of at least some of our elected federal officeholders regarding the need to change the way chronic care is delivered if there are to be cost savings and better care at the same time. Advocates of change, such as the editorial board of the *New York Times*, recognized in the editorial at the end of 2009—"The Case for Reform"—the link between how medical and hospital care is delivered and why costs continue to increase, particularly for the elderly.

> The inexorably rising cost of hospital and medical care is the underlying factor that drives up premiums, deductibles and co-payments. No one yet has an answer to the problem. But the bill would launch an array of pilot projects to test new payments and health care delivery systems

within Medicare. These include, for example, incentives to coordinate hospital and post-hospital care to head off needless readmissions, better coordination of care for the chronically Ill, and incentives for doctors to provide a patient's total care for a flat fee instead of charging for each test or service provided. (p. A26)

All of these potentially valuable improvements in the quality of care delivered are based on putting patients first. In many respects this expanded emphasis on chronic care as person-centered care is a sharp rebuke to the way medicine in America is organized and how it delivers care. One of the most articulate advocates of person centered care, Allen B. Barbour, former head of the Division of General Internal Medicine and chief of the Stanford University Medical College's Diagnostic Clinic, put the person first and sought to see the situation in which that person was encountered. Therefore, the emphasis is on clinical judgment regarding the patient rather than diagnosis. It follows, contrary to common practices in health care, that there is a critical need for mutual involvement on the part of the physician and the patient in determining the healing process.

Dr. Barbour offers a critique of the medical model and the fact that there is little connection in the practice of health care with the patient's personal life. His book, *Caring for Patients* (1995), advocates that the work of doctors is dealing with the distress undergone by patients rather than simply fighting disease. Susan Sontag and other cancer patients would take notice of this approach but would still want to get good disease fighters on their side.

Community-based care, as the following chapters will show, is clearly a quality-of-life benefit for patients with serious chronic illnesses. Health care system builders and providers are starting to look for financial incentives for helping patients learn how to live with chronic illnesses. This kind of thinking fits the demographics of an aging population whose members often need guidance on what risks to avoid and what kinds of information they require to survive with diseases that will be with them their entire lives.

Chronic illness care has arrived on the national agenda, a way of showing that it is a high priority and not just a wish for the future. The legislative process of creating the legal foundation for health care reform was started by the House of Representatives Committees on Ways and Means, Energy and Commerce, and Education and Labor and finally offered for consideration by the entire House by Speaker Nancy Pelosi on October 29, 2009. This yearlong effort provides a glimpse, through a detailed summary created by the three principal committees, at how serious the members of this legislative body were about dealing with chronic illness in a more effective way. Under sections of the bill creating Medicare reforms, there are payment incentives established for hospitals and post-acute care providers to discourage preventable hospital admissions. Another section of the proposed law called for bundling payments that encourage providers to coordinate patient care across the entire complement of services, starting in the doctor's office, through the hospital stay and perhaps a rehabilitative or nursing home admission, and then back to home. The original House bill (HR 3962) also included funding to create a pilot program to reward providers who agree to furnish services necessary to make their practices medical homes. The medical home will encourage full access to patients and supply coordinated and comprehensive care.

Similar financial incentives are created for providers in the Medicaid delivery system, the federal-state program for the poor and medically indigent in the United States. Payments through Medicaid for primary care would be increased to match at 100 percent of Medicare rates starting in 2012, with the federal government paying 100 percent of the increased costs from 2012 through 2014 and 90 percent thereafter. (At the time I write these optimistic words about support for primary care, Congress in August 2010 has still not made the appropriations to support Medicaid in an enriched way.) This is clearly a step in the right direction when it comes to ending the two-tier system of care in the United States, with Medicaid beneficiaries having to find doctors who will accept the lower remuneration, even in states that are generous, compared to other states, but not compared to Medicare or what commercial insurance pays for a primary care visit. Medicaid payments nationally are 74 percent of Medicare payments for the same procedure and consequently some physicians are starting to refuse Medicaid beneficiaries because they cost medical practices too much to deliver the service and it is becoming more difficult to cross-fund or make up the difference in revenues (Sack, 2010, p. A1).

While rightwing critics of reform decry the cost of making these changes in financing, there is no way that health care can be improved in the United States without spending for underfunded programs. Therefore, there are several platforms in the bill for launching new initiatives. These efforts strike out at the cost and ineffectiveness of chronic care in the United States. A five-year pilot program would support a large-scale evaluation of medical-home models for beneficiaries, including medically fragile children. This pilot program is robustly funded, making available $1.235 billion from federal sources.

These elements of delivery system reform that ultimately made it into PPACA are a result of widespread recognition among legislators that the health care system is broken when it comes to chronic care. Usually, the problem, fueled by the lack of community-based care, leads to unnecessary hospitalization and rehospitalization. This effort at delivery system reform is both good for consumers and is also a way to reduce national health care expenses since per diem costs for hospital care are major contributors to our soaring medical expenditures.

While there are some excellent models for reinventing chronic care, they are few and far between. Most doctors do not want to take the financial risk of introducing these innovations without guidance along with financial incentives. Helping to solve the problem is Don Klitgaard, MD, a primary care physician at the Myrtus Medical Center in Harlan, Iowa. Using the medical home model, Kiltgaard and his colleagues have reorganized primary care to follow the medical home approach. Patients with health problems are tracked closely by clinic nurses so that if they detect that a patient is no longer in a stable condition, he or she will be sent to the emergency department, even in the middle of the night (Alonzo-Zaldivar, 2009).

A medical home program should be adept at preventing readmissions to hospitals as well as keeping people out of emergency departments. Twenty percent of Medicare patients who are discharged from the hospital are readmitted within 30 days of discharge, often a result of poor care coordination, the incompatibility of prescribed medications, or failure to instruct patients on how to manage their condition following discharge (Minot, 2009, p. 4).

The failure to supply care coordination helps to explain why there is waste in the system. Dr. Klitgaard knows, as well as many other advocates for delivery system change, that "three-fourths of Medicare's budget goes to less than one-fourth of its clients, usually patients with five or more chronic conditions, such as diabetes, heart failure or lung disease. They average 14 different doctors a year. Some juggle dozens of prescriptions" (Alonzo-Zaldivar, 2009). With 83 percent of the Medicare population with at least one chronic disease, disease management and, more importantly, care coordination become the essential ingredients in delivering services to senior citizens and younger individuals who have disabilities so severe that they cannot support themselves through work (Anderson, 2005). Clearly, there needs to be some rethinking as to how to make a difference in health care for the chronically ill.

How can this situation be corrected? Much of chronic care needs to be rebalanced to encourage more efficiency and effectiveness. To end the unnecessary visits to the wrong specialists, avoid duplicative tests, get the right medications, and reduce the likelihood of uncontrolled health problems, we need more medical homes. Preventing the worst complications of diabetes, for example, including blindness, can make both for a better quality of life for the consumer and rein in expenditures for the health care delivery system.

Dr. Klitgaard has found that not only has the medical home approach improved patient satisfaction but that before the program was implemented at the Harlan clinic, fewer patients had control over their high blood pressure and blood sugar levels. However, both clinicians and health policy analysts wonder whether this bold legislation will do enough to attract newly minted doctors to primary care and create financial incentives for providers to deliver care coordination services, monitoring, and educating patients about their serious chronic illnesses. Medical school debt, being the burden that it is, helps to encourage medical college graduates to seek out residencies in specialties that can lead to practices that can generate incomes that can help pay off that debt in a reasonable period of time. Encouraging entry into primary care can help change the way medical care is organized.

Delivery system change can also affect patient behavior in ways that are helpful to the patient. Some delivery systems that are supported by financing that allows doctors to hire nurses to be available to answer questions from patients with serious chronic illnesses have seen patients become willing to call a nurse where they would be reluctant to attempt to reach a doctor (Abelson, 2010a, p. B7).

The momentum for remaking chronic care is found both in the public and the private sectors of health care financing. States, through health care foundations started with funds returned by Blue Cross and Blue Shield Insurers that went for-profit, such as the NYS Health Foundation, are now advocating through comprehensive reports that there are options for saving money and improving care through expanding primary care to provide for the chronically ill, creating accountable care organizations (perhaps the next big thing) that integrate hospital and community care, and financing such care through bundled payments (Lewin Group, 2010).

Even insurance companies are starting to get into the act via attempts at getting the attention of beneficiaries to shift to value in health care. An innovative program in Oregon is starting to lay off more of the costs of knee replacements, hysterectomies, and heart-bypass surgery to the patient and picking up more of the costs of the treatment of diabetes and depression because the results are better (Appleby, 2010, p. B1). This slick approach leaves the discretionary procedures, often costly but not life saving, in the hands of the patient as they decide whether it is worth the price to them when there are alternatives that can produce good outcomes health-wise. Not every knee needs to be replaced when there are some aches and pains and going without surgery may encourage patients to take advantage of coordinated care for diabetes.

Finally, we find support for the medical-home model in high government places. The strongest professional advocates for the medical home, the American Academy of Family Physicians, received strong backing for the concept in 2008 from then candidate Barack Obama, who in responding to the association's query said, "I support the concept of a patient centered medical home" and when he becomes president he would "encourage and provide appropriate payment for providers who implement the medical home model" (Wikipedia, 2009). The implementation of this promise, beginning in 2010, supplies the backdrop for our travels through the land of chronic care.

None of these stubborn facts about the way the U.S. health care delivery system is distorted would have been established if it was not for efforts begun following the creation in 1965 of the monumental programs Medicare and Medicaid. The critique of U.S. health care was begun by a small cadre of reform-minded doctors, epidemiologists, and public health experts, who did not depended on receiving fees from patients for services or the blessings of local, state, and national medical associations to maintain their livelihoods. Because of their relative freedom from being dependent on fee-for-service financing and their commitment to seek quality health care at a reasonable cost for all, they were willing to speak truth to power. The recognition of this maverick group goes back almost 40 years. Designated by sociologist Robert Alford the "corporate rationalizers" (1972), these research- and policy-minded professionals continued to make the case for systemic change in the financing and delivery of health services in the United States. Making the rational real—the Left Wing interpretation of the philosophy of Hegel, the nineteenth-century German powerhouse—is the origin of Alford's name for these active promoters of a more just and affordable health care system.

Still there needs to be energetic and articulate leadership from the medical profession if the vast remaking of the health care system, as well as the movement to universal coverage, is to be accomplished. We need to quickly close the gap between what the policy wonks think needs to be done and what knowledge the general public requires to legitimate the changes being established through the PPACA. Elliot Fisher, Donald Berwick, and Karen Davis got it right when in the June 11, 2009 issue of the *New England Journal of Medicine* they said that physicians can become our most credible and effective leaders of progress toward a new world of coordinated, sensible, outcome-oriented care in which they and their communities will be far better off (p. 3). But how does that happen when we face a deep divide between the experts concerned with cost savings and integrated delivery systems and a public wounded by either the burden of costly medical bills or lack of access to care because they are uninsured? Many Americans distrust the educated elite and confuse them with those with real power in the United States, the owners of our corporations.

This is a great challenge to the members of the profession and the organizations that represent medicine, both to government and to corporations. To date, the profession of medicine has not made a concerted effort to teach the public that there are priorities within the world of health care. In a country built around a strong belief that "what's in it for me" rules all priorities this may be a hard sell. Still, there is good reason to believe that the public is educable. Consider how successful seat-belt laws have been in promoting compliance (and saving lives). For a long time, policy experts believed that only passive restraints made sense because they believed that Americans would not take to buckling up.

The same thing applies to other forms of learning, including recognition that there are times when heroic interventions are useless. Doctors have learned how to teach patients' relatives and friends when to withdraw life supports. Medicine must be the guardian of medical resources because few other professions, public officials, or consumers have the knowledge to make choices about when to end the life of a person on a dying trajectory.

More abstract, but equally important, are efforts to provide population-based health care, a form of prioritizing whereby physicians in a particular area determine the health care needs of the community based on demographic and epidemiological data. To treat asthma effectively, for example, doctors have to know where the highest risk for the disease resides in the community, not just treat the most easily accessible. Treatment also involves family education to help keep patients with asthma well and out of hospital care.

Consumers and patients would listen more closely to what doctors and health policy experts say about prioritizing the use of scarce resources if more respect and admiration were expressed for the profession. There is a strong need to institutionally retain the essence of why young people become physicians to serve society and humankind. This altruism needs to be maintained through the careers of physicians and not be lost once medical school is completed and residencies acquired. Expressions of continuing caring and compassion will generate respect for the advice the profession gives and will provide public legitimacy to the prioritizing of health care needs. Thus there is a practical side to idealism and we need to take advantage of it.

Some of that respect could be recaptured (eventually) if physicians volunteered their time and sat on community advisory boards related to health care services and the provision of other public goods. They need to hear directly from laypeople what their needs are and not to quickly cut them off when they speak because they think they received the message, as they often do when in face-to-face contact with a patient prior to an examination. While there is no time now to go back to the community before the big decisions are made in Congress, since our legislators have already acted, this pledge of concern can be a commitment made during the public occasions when physicians go out and attempt to explain to the public why certain reforms are necessary to promote the common good.

Moreover, the profession of medicine needs to become imbued with a spirit of partnership, one that can help improve quality and increase access and delivery of services at more modest costs. This willingness to partner with other constituent groups in the field of health care could be done if other groups acquired the same spirit. Working out a structure of cooperation through partnership means that neither government nor corporations gain the upper hand in controlling health care. A balance between government intervention and profit making has to occur so that the rights of patients and professionals are respected. I foresee the various players, especially the insurance companies, being regulated much as public utilities rather than as unfettered corporations.

Along with the creation of regulated corporations that sell insurance and offer managed care plans, there will also be a concerted public health effort to create a foundation of prevention, based on the recognition within the Public Health Service of the U.S. Department of Health and Human Services (HHS), that diseases such as diabetes, heart disease, and cancer are implicated in 7 out of 10 deaths in the United States and explain why health care costs are out of control since they account for 75 percent of the national spending on health care.

The Public Health Service is out in front on the issue of primary prevention of chronic illness rather than management, but it is a start. The Healthy People initiative, launched on December 2, 2010, has recognized that improvement in the lives of our citizens depends on preventing the onset of serious chronic illnesses. Following a thorough listening time, involving suggestions and criticisms from multiple government officials, 2,000 organizations, as well as the public, a comprehensive set of objectives has been drafted. There are now innovative approaches being encouraged by the U.S. Department of Health and Human Services through the "myHealthyPeople" (www .healthypeople.gov/2020/default.aspx) applications, permitting communities to track their progress in reducing the incidence of chronic diseases with reachable targets for health improvement.

Finally, there is a platform to build on for physicians who are blind to the larger realities of population health and the need for integrated delivery systems. Foundation support and federal funding have created a wealth of information about the shortfalls in chronic care in the United States in the twenty-first century. With the help of the current generation of researchers, system planners, and policy wonks, and patients as well, I will first examine the depth of the problem, starting with the characteristics of our aging population, before moving on to the current financing and delivery of chronic care in the United States.

# 1

# Demographic Destinies

We live in a remarkable age of scientific discovery, and there are major possibilities now and in the near future for the transformation of how health care is delivered. It is no small wonder that the human genome project has fascinated both scientists and laypeople around the world; new interventions are discovered almost weekly that can potentially identify or, even better, neutralize a gene that is disease related. Nevertheless, there are few practical interventions that have emerged as a result of the project. Some discoveries suggest that treatments work, e.g., for breast cancer, when a gene is present or absent. This revolution in discovery will lead to a reinvention of medical specialties and many of the current fields, such as internal medicine, will become part of genetics. Disease has become part of virtual reality since it is part of an elaborate code, one written by nature and not a programmer in Silicon Valley. Consequently, medical education and postdoctoral training will be less relevant to patient care if it does not absorb the theoretical and practical aspects of genetics.

While we can get carried away with the idea that genes appear to shape our destinies, there is another, older paradigm that is in operation in looking at health and illness. When it comes to understanding the origins of differential rates of chronic diseases and mortality in different societies—or even the same society—there are strong indications that physical and social environmental factors play a large role. The way we live now and how these patterns are arrived at and change help to explain the current risks of chronic diseases and mortality more than the extremely slow rate of change found in genetic evolution. Moreover, it is possible that environmental factors trigger genetic predispositions.

We may be living longer, but old age comes with baggage, a kind of graying of the United States that was first identified in the 1970s. I anticipate that marketing experts will be making us well aware of this shift in demographics. The corporate sponsorship of national shuffleboard competitions should increase tenfold. Population change creates markets that were never conceived of a century ago. By the year 2030, one third of the population of the United States will be 50 years old or older, with 70 million Americans turning 65 between 2010 and the magic year of 2030 (Freudenheim, 2010, p. D6). And this growth of the older adult population of this country, as well as others, will occur despite the fact that we do not have the life expectancy of other advanced industrialized countries such as Japan. Even within the population cohort 50 years old and older, there are sharp differences in life chances due to lifestyle differences and risks found in the environment. There is wide variation in opportunities in our society and there are wide variations in getting the help one needs to overcome illness. The knowledge base that has emerged in the study of public health and epidemiology has shown that some interventions in a relatively short period of time can reduce the disparities in life expectancy. The United States Public Health Service has committed itself to reducing the health disparities and access to health care between people of differing socioeconomic status, those with or without disabilities, and the various ethnic groups in this country, including all age cohorts.

The graying of the United States also means that there are opportunities as well as problems to master, if we act now, and create the number of nurses and doctors in the appropriate specialties, e.g., geriatrics, to care for a segment of the population that is going to challenge the existing health care system. While geriatrics is a specialty, it is still a close cousin of primary care since many of the patients seen by these doctors and nurses will be residing in the community and need appropriate care to retain their independence. Maintenance of independence, a key condition for a happy old age, is a condition that requires preparation and planning on the national, state, and local levels as well as by the individual and within intergenerational families.

The potential is there for a healthy tomorrow, to borrow a slogan from the United States Public Health Service's campaign for better health care for children. Even the disparities found in life expectancy and health disparities in comparisons between rich and poor countries could be narrowed. The implication is that social remedies can reduce the disparities that epidemiologists, demographers, and public health specialists find between rich and poor countries. Some of these differences are so huge that it is hard to believe they exist.

These comparisons are based on large data sets, collected and analyzed over long periods of time. Life expectancy differences between rich and poor countries, according to Michael Marmot, a leading British epidemiologist, can be as much as an astounding 48 years! And within a country, the spread between rich and poor in terms of life expectancy can be as much as 20 years (Marmot, 2005). Reversing the odds is possible, often with the use of some inexpensive and quickly distributed equipment and supplies. Dramatic changes in life expectancy and the debilitating effects of serious illness (e.g., malaria) can be quite dramatic when even low cost and low technology efforts (e.g., bed nets to fight malaria) are made to prevent disease. Improvements in growing techniques and irrigation can generate better crop yields and reduce hunger-related deaths in many parts of the world that suffer from a limited food supply for a growing population related to weak harvests and frequent drought.

Health disparities can account for differences in mortality, not just when countries are compared but even when the workforce differences of large organizations are deployed to predict the chances of mortality. Most recently, Stringhini and her colleagues (2010) analyzed the data from the 1985 British Whitehall II longitudinal study which followed for many years more than 10,000 civil servants ages 35 to 55 to determine whether health behaviors contributed to the disparities in mortality rates between the high-ranking and lower-ranking government employees. The National Health Service in the United Kingdom makes access to services equal regardless of income, education, or occupation so that differences in death rates cannot be explained by limits on access to medical services.

The less well off and the better off act in ways that produce or limit risks to health. In this London-based population, there was an association between socioeconomic position and mortality, with most of the differences accounted for by differences in health behaviors. In commenting on this research report, James H. Dunn (2010) suggested that from birth on, "the stress pathway is partly a behavioral pathway and unhealthy behaviors are coping mechanisms for the stress of low socioeconomic status" (p. 1199). In this narrative, Dunn also argues that the failure of some low-socioeconomic individuals to develop self-regulation and executive function skills may discourage them from competing for more valued socioeconomic positions (p. 1200). So it is not only health that is made vulnerable by poor coping skills;

also the opportunity to advance is put into question by the absence of skills essential for certain high-level bureaucratic positions.

Strangely, it is astounding that even when the incidence of a disease or morbidity is the same in different socioeconomic classes, the death rate may be higher for those lower on the social ladder (Mackenbach et al., 2008). Limited access to resources and lifestyle differences may pose certain risk factors for the lower strata. Some of these risks are immediate, e.g., inconsistency in receiving appropriate number of calories for a given age may mean missing school days. There may be long-term consequences as well from early exposure to stress. Indeed, exposure to childhood poverty has been shown to be associated with increased morbidity or sickness in adult life, e.g., diabetes, as well as increased mortality, including death from unintentional injuries and homicide (Galobardes, Lunch, and Smith, 2008).

These results are not limited to the United Kingdom. Similar findings were reported recently when chronic conditions and health status were assessed in the United States and the poor and non-poor are compared. When a cross-section of Americans 55 and older was interviewed, health status for these age groups varied internally by income. Schoenborn and Heyman (2009) note that "[p]oor adults and adults with Medicaid were the most disadvantaged in terms of health status, physical and social functioning health care utilization, and health behaviors." Whatever the risk for poor health, including selected chronic conditions, difficulties with physical and social impairments, and behaviors such as smoking, the poor and near poor were more likely than the nonpoor to assess their health as poor or fair rather than good or excellent. It has been shown that while some of the impoverished Americans, with the least in the way of resources, may remain bright-sided, the majority among the disinherited take a darker view of their situation.

Based on these findings, the John D. and Catherine T. MacArthur Foundation is currently supporting a prospective study of the impact of housing on the cardiovascular health of Latinos in the Bronx. The award, to Albert Einstein College of Medicine, will permit Dr. Earle Chambers and his colleagues to "determine if those who live in mixed income housing by way of government housing vouchers have lower cardiovascular risk than those who live in either government-subsidized public housing developments or in unsubsidized housing" (Einstein, 2010, p. 1). The MacArthur Foundation is supporting 13 similar projects throughout the United States with nearly $6 million in grants. All of these projects will measure stress levels as well as

**Table 1.1  Percentage of Adults 65 Years Old and Older with Selected Health Conditions and Impairments (2004–2007)**

|          | Vision Impairment | Hypertension | Heart Disease | Hearing Impairment |
|----------|-------------------|--------------|---------------|--------------------|
| 65–74    | 13.5              | 50.8         | 26.8          | 30.9               |
| 75–84    | 18.3              | 55.7         | 35.3          | 43.7               |
| 85 plus  | 26.9              | 54.3         | 40.7          | 62.1               |

*Source:* From Schoenborn and Heyman, 2009.

introduce measures related to the hazards and dangers found in the urban environments involved in this multisite study.

Class differences do matter since they affect life chances, and seen through the eyes of conservative members of the U.S. Congress and talk-show hosts on the radio, any discussion of social stratification is identified as divisive. The fact remains that this is an important subject for discussion if we are to have a democratic country. As Issacs and Schroeder (2004) put it, "what data exist show a consistent inverse and stepwise relationship between class and premature death" (p. 1137). Pretending that social classes do not exist in our country because of our one-person-one-vote political system does not lead to action to redistribute resources to bridge these gaps. Nor do I think that many Republican members of Congress are eager to trade places with members of the underclass to prove that social classes do not exist in the United States.

Age, more obviously, also makes a difference when it comes to the prevalence of disease. Beyond the age of 65, according to data from the 2004 to 2007 reports of the National Health Interview Surveys, the common chronic conditions—heart disease and hypertension— increase dramatically, particularly when the age range is broken down into 10-year intervals. Functional impairments such as vision and hearing loss increase even more dramatically with aging (see Table 1.1). This way of presenting chronic conditions leaves out cancer, a disease that is common among senior citizens. However, some of the deficits or impairments listed here are subject to remediation via technology.

While age is often associated with the onset of disease, it does not explain why some individuals become victims of chronic illness and others do not. We have some leads or clues on how to explain this mystery. Public policies can have health consequences. When Prime Minister Margaret Thatcher led the Conservatives' charge against big

government, individuals in Great Britain who were subject to privatization at their place of employment were considered both exposed to
new stresses and subjects worthy of research attention. This unusual
situation produced an opportunity for a prospective or follow-up
study of current and former white-collar civil servants, with varying
degrees of job security. Ferrie et al. (2001) analyzed the data on the
comparative risks for longstanding illness or poor mental health
according to employment status. The securely employed had far lower
risks of acquiring these conditions than did the insecurely employed
or the unemployed. In fact, the insecurely employed were far more
likely than the other groups to suffer from poor mental health. The
Great Recession of 2008–10 (and perhaps beyond) creates the same
kind of natural experiment for epidemiologists for follow-up studies.
Research suggests that economic downturns, which happen periodically, provide a sound justification for universal health coverage,
organized and available through a social insurance option such as
Medicare, that won't disappear if businesses go under or when benefits are shrunk because of efforts on the part of entrepreneurs to save
money.

Despite the commonsense view that bad economic conditions are
harmful to our health, the report of the United States Centers for Disease Control and Prevention's National Center on Health Statistics cal-
culated that life expectancy at birth in 2007, just before the economic
downturn, increased 2.5 months and was up to 78 years from 77.7 in
the prior year. Even for those who were born 70 to 80 years ago, the
leading sources of morbidity and mortality—heart disease and
cancer—account for fewer deaths. Overall, fewer people in these contemporary times died from heart disease–related problems such as
stroke, diabetes, and high blood pressure (Xu, Kochanek, and Tejada-
Vera, 2009). Clearly, there is another sound justification for Medicare
to cover chronic care more adequately in the community rather than
in hospital care than it does now to align itself with the increased longevity within the population.

## BRAVE NEW OPTIONS

Improvements in life expectancy, especially when the dreaded disease
cancer is the subject of conversation, are to some extent the result of
early detection and treatment. New treatments for cancer are precise
because drugs can be designed for particular kinds of cancer. As a
result of these advances, the popular cultural view on cancer has

changed from what the late novelist and political essayist Norman Mailer once called "cancer gulch" on a television talk show to a more hopeful perception of the disease. Even the advertisements for cancer treatment centers found in newspapers, on television, and on the Internet express the narrative that cancer is left behind by most people who get care at that center. There is also the ever-growing popular belief that if you survive long enough, there will be a new drug that will become available widely making cure possible. Consider the impact this has on people willingly writing a living will. Why not be kept alive, even in a vegetative state, if some new wonder drug might come along and, like the kiss of the prince in a fairy tale, make you whole again? However, the bridge to a cure may not be the most secure one to walk on, and extreme measures to prolong life may not be pleasant.

There are some other considerations when it comes to extending life when an acute condition can be transformed into a chronic illness. If cure is not possible, containment could occur, much in the way that AIDS has become a chronic disease because there are therapies that were once in the pipeline that now limit the severity of the condition.

Most stories of the treatment of life-threatening disease focus on how bravely people cope when powerful and often experimental therapies are introduced. Receiving treatment, for many, is not without often-debilitating consequences that can make living an enormously painful struggle. There are stories of brave cancer victims that serve as inspirations to others with the disease. Amy Dockser Marcus, a health beat reporter for the *Wall Street Journal*, won the Pulitzer Prize in 2005 for her 2004 series of articles on confronting the curse of cancer. However, seeking cures may not always be all that it is cracked up to be. A 41-year-old woman with breast cancer, given only a 5 percent chance of survival, had a mastectomy and other surgeries and underwent chemotherapy. As a consequence, there were such serious chronic health problems that her heart failed and she underwent a heart transplant, which in turn had negative consequences. Beyond the medications to keep her body from rejecting the new heart, there were serious interpersonal concerns, previously below the surface, that emerged when she and her husband discovered that they had different coping styles. There was also the problem of what to tell the children and how often she could be there for them (Marcus, 2004c).

Marcus goes on in other brilliant articles to suggest that we are at a frontier of transformation in the treatment of cancer, and if you are a recent victim of that disease, there is hope that a cure will be found in the near future. New approaches to using surgery to aggressively treat lung cancer can make a difference in survival. By the end of the article, which follows the four-year path of treatment for an ex-smoker and mother of two teenage daughters who is first diagnosed with lung cancer at 41, we find a reversal of conventional medical wisdom so that a National Cancer Institute report, quoted by Ms. Marcus, stated that "The stigma that lung cancer is a self-inflicted disease, coupled with a pervasive sense of therapeutic nihilism conspires to create a medical environment in which many patients with advanced cancer are not even offered treatment." Surgery combined with targeted drug therapy can limit the growth of tumors, according to researchers at such august sites as New York City's Memorial Sloan-Kettering Hospital (Marcus, 2004a).

Treatments "outside of the box" have other consequences. All of this effort, at the frontiers of knowledge about treatment of advanced lung cancer, where patients were given a 5 percent chance of living a few months, has lead to patients and their providers asking painful and provocative questions related to whether powerful doses of toxic chemotherapy treatments were necessary as compared to less toxic treatments. Needless to say, through the power of second guessing, the results showed that the less toxic treatments were adequate in limiting tumor growth. Drug trials do deal with toxicity on healthy subjects and this may underrepresent the impact on people with cancer or other systemic diseases.

While it can be said that the trend over time with regard to longevity is in the right direction, there is room for improvement in expanding life expectancy, given the countries with which we are compared. The United States sits sadly behind other countries "in life expectancy and preventable deaths from diseases like diabetes, circulatory problems and respiratory issues like asthma" (Harris, 2008, p. 2). These diseases require chronic care interventions, which, incredibly, are often not available in a country that spends $6,714 per person annually—almost twice what other countries spend on health care. Reductions in death rates from chronic diseases will only mean that more persistent care will be required, starting at an earlier age than in the past. It is anticipated that the race for the cure will be run with more thought behind treatment decisions than in the past. Hopefully, effective but inexpensive low-tech solutions will be available and they will crowd out the expensive high-tech solutions that don't work or are of equal efficacy. Less can be more but readers can rest assured that manufacturers of these expensive solutions will continue to argue that they help some people, if not everybody. More importantly, coordination of care from many specialty providers is a high priority that needs to be attained.

## SOCIETY AND POPULATION

There is a theoretic and empirical connection to our current dilemma. The proliferation of conditions that require chronic care begins with the transition from societies that are characterized by high birth rates and high death rates to societies that have reduced the death rate via economic growth and environmental improvements (housing, sanitation, clean water) while the birth rate remains high. With children born into industrialized societies living longer, both at birth and later in life, there is an increase, along with the population, in the incidence of chronic diseases and a reduction in infectious diseases. Furthermore, in advanced industrial societies, with a reduced birth rate, the population is older. With fewer children to compete with, the old grow even older, and there are more of us now than at any previous point in American history. However, with age comes wisdom, or so it is said, *and* chronic illness, and surely the need for chronic care. In a dual sense, now and in the near future, chronic care comes of age.

The shift in population is also instructive in determining whether medicine as a profession is equipped both culturally and structurally to deal with chronic illnesses. Medicine in the United States, in particular, became recognized as the major profession responsible not by offering care for chronic illness but through public health improvements and technological developments that made acute care more effective. First, there was the invention of anesthesia, which permitted surgeons to operate without having to deal with the bothersome patient. In addition, it was far easier to teach surgery when the patient was unconscious, and so the surgical theaters, made famous by the Philadelphia artist Thomas Eakins in his 1889 painting, *The Agnew Clinic*, showed the drama of learning how to perform a decisive intervention. Preventing wound infection during and after surgery by following rules regarding hand washing and using large quantities of antiseptic fluids also helped promote survival. Second, the X-ray machine made locating bone fractures more precise and therefore treating the break was made more effective. Finally, a half a century later, the invention and use of antibiotics such as penicillin meant that systemic infections could be treated. Some major persistent diseases of the nineteenth century, such as tuberculosis, were all but eliminated until new strains of the bacteria began to emerge in the late twentieth century.

The model for involvement on the part of physicians and patients was one of activity and passivity, respectively. Follow-up of patients was usually not necessary since instruction was not required and the patched-up patients went back to their pursuits prior to the intervention. The discovery of insulin as a lifelong treatment for diabetes was one of the first bases for the guidance-cooperation model. Still, demographic change in the population will require paying attention to the social side of aging at the same time that medical problems are addressed. Policies to make that happen need to be formulated now and not wait until the next century when American society will be much older. Forward-thinking policy does not appear to be an American forte and our practices are often suspected of being less valuable to consumers and payers than they could be. Many private insurance payers have little to gain by looking closely at what they pay for since they simply pass on the increases in costs to employers who create group plans or to buyers in the individual health insurance market.

Alas, the overall health of the U.S. population, despite leading the world in per capita expenditures on health care, is often considered less than adequate when universally accepted major population indicators, such as infant mortality, are compared. In 1960, the United States ranked 12th in the world when infant mortality was compared with other countries. By 2006, the infant mortality rate, while dropping in the United States, remained well above other industrialized countries that also improved. According to data released by the Centers for Disease Control and Prevention, the ranking of the United States dropped further to 29th. An increase in preterm births, particularly among African American women, appears to account for a substantial part of the persistently high infant mortality rate (Harris, 2008, p. 1).

The risks to children of death and disease do not end at birth. High death rates for preschool children have been linked with living in a household with relative income poverty. There is an ecologic relationship between the rate of child poverty in a country and the death rate for children under the age of five. Countries that implement redistributive income policies that supply benefits for families of young children, such as Sweden and Norway, have the lowest percentage of children living in poverty and the lowest death rates for children five and younger per 1,000 children in the population (Emerson, 2009). This is a robust foundation for taking care of oneself later on in life. The food-stamp program initiated in the United States in the 1970s has reduced the possibility that hunger will be a major problem during the large and persistent economic downturn that started in 2007.

Nevertheless, our population as the populations of many technologically advanced societies (e.g., as in Japan where by 2100 half the population will be ages 60 years or older) will show an increasing percentage of elderly within it. While we are still 90 years away from reaching 2100 or the "Aging Century," as it has already been labeled, there are still many concerns about rising medical expenditures due to an aging U.S. population (Landefeld, Winker, and Chernof, 2009, p. 2703).

Planning for health care for an older population would start, logically, with increasing the number of physicians who are learned in geriatrics, the medical specialty that focuses on the elderly. Currently, while Medicare supports the training of physicians in various specialties, it does not demand that core content in geriatrics be required (Landefeld, Winker, and Chernof, 2009, p. 2703). The medical school curricula, according to my physician colleagues, is well defended by the professoriat and sometimes is not aligned with actual clinical practice.

It is a disgrace that U.S. medical schools are not any more forward thinking. They seem to be prepared to require courses that support subspecialties rather than more general specialties such as geriatrics. Dr. Christine K. Cassel (2009), the editor of the *Journal of the American Medical Association*, strongly suggests it is time for a change because "in each year from 2007 to 2009 fewer than 100 US medical graduates pursued postdoctoral training in geriatrics" (p. 2701). This recruitment to geriatrics hardly comes close to meeting the demand.

Without more geriatricians, there cannot be a personalized, i.e., patient-centered care system that primary-care advocates say we need to meet the challenge of an aging century and the years leading up to it. The movement to patient-centered care means that the objectification of patients will be challenged both at the bedside and, more importantly, by providers listening to what individuals combating chronic diseases want in the way of treatment and instruction on how to take care of themselves. Older people are not the only patients of concern when it comes to attempts at personalizing care, as can be seen when families are affected by serious chronic illnesses in children.

## CHILDREN AND THE GROWTH AMONG THEM OF CHRONIC ILLNESS

Despite the strong emphasis on the need for more geriatricians found among the critics of the planners of medical education, there is also recognition among those who do research on the health of children that the numbers are increasing when it comes to chronic illness. A recent report on the rates of obesity and other childhood chronic conditions among children and youth indicates that three cohorts of children, followed from 1988 to 2006, indicated that there were changes in the prevalence of chronic conditions during these decades. While the number of existing cases increased from the beginning of one cohort study to the other, there was a trend toward a dynamic count, with some children and youth starting out with a condition, e.g., obesity, and losing it six years later, and some children first surveyed becoming chronically ill later during the period of observation. The results on childhood prevalence of obesity revealed a shocking increase—the rates more than doubled from 12.8 percent in 1994 to 26.6 percent in 2006 (Van Cleave, Gortmaker, and Perrin, 2010). Some have declared the rise as one of epidemic proportions.

In commenting on the results of this study in an editorial in the *Journal of the American Medical Association*, Neal Halfon and Paul Newacheck (2010), two recognized experts on child health, attempted to account for the sharp jump by listing improvements of the survival rates among those children with chronic illnesses, better access to care and new methods for diagnosing chronic conditions, especially in the emotional and behavior categories. They observed that

> Increasing rates of obesity appear to be driving the overall trend in prevalence described by Van Cleave et al, but significant increases were noted for all physical health conditions, with lesser increases for asthma and fairly minimal changes in the reported rates of learning and behavioral problems. (p. 665)

The good news was that some conditions did resolve, although the authors of the study that used data from the National Longitudinal Survey of Youth also indicated that there was no way to determine from the data that were analyzed which children were likely to lose their obesity or go into remission with regard to another chronic condition.

While I note that remissions do occur in children and infant mortality obviates the need for chronic care services for those usually poor victims, often there are those who survive in the United States with serious chronic illnesses who need coordinated treatment and family support. Conditions that start in childhood help to contribute to the rates of chronic disease among older adults as well as those who are young and middle aged. The next chapter will look closely at various prevalent chronic diseases and the kind of care they require.

# 2

# Chronic Illness in America Today

Even without President Obama's ringing endorsement of patient-centered medical homes, the evidence is strong that chronic illness care is a major problem that needs to be addressed. Our aging population not only means that there will be fewer contributors to Social Security and Medicare in the work force, but there will also be far more people living with one or more chronic illnesses, which may be an indication that people are living longer. Not only are there more people who report that they have a chronic illness—44 percent in 2005—but there are more people reporting that they suffer from more than one condition. The evidence for this statement comes from the last Medical Expenditure Panel Survey (MEPS), an annual national data collection effort that not only tells us about health conditions among the people sampled but also, as the title of the survey indicates, how much is spent and what sources these expenditures come from. MEPS is a good barometer of where payments were derived and where they go, although it does not tell us much about the quality of care received. Nevertheless, spending is a way of measuring what are the most prevalent diseases of an aging society. We also utilize a health care delivery system that needs to deliver better services at least cost and see the results in reductions in the incidents and prevalence rates of disease as well as consequent disabilities that accompany serious chronic illnesses.

Costs in health care will only increase as the U.S. population ages and if the current patterns of spending hold. Most of us will not go comfortably into old age and we will need all the help we can get. At this point, women constitute 58 percent of the population age 65 and older and men 42 percent. In a recent analysis of the 2004 national health care expenditures by gender, it has been reported that women in general spend more on health care than men. When the elderly were compared according to gender, women accounted for 61 percent of health care spending for people age 65 and older. "Per capita, elderly women's spending was 12 percent more than their male counterparts" (Cylus, Hartman, Washington, Andrews, and Catlin, 2010, p. 6). Overall, per capita spending for women 65 and older was three times greater than for women 19 to 64; and for men, the expenditures per capita for those 65 and older compared with men 19 to 64 was 3.6 times greater (Cylus, Hartman, Washington, Andrews, and Catlin, 2010, p. 5). The presence and treatment of chronic illness in an aging society does lead to unsustainable expenditures.

Before I proceed with more specific evidence that chronic conditions account for most of our health care expenditures, particularly through Medicare, it is important to recognize that concern about whether the U.S. health care delivery system can address the issues related to chronic care go back to the 1970s, when the full impact of Medicare access was being identified by health policy analysts who sought a more rational delivery system. William Glazier, writing in the *Scientific American* in 1973, summarized the problem well and was prophetic:

> The medical system encounters several types of problems in dealing with the chronically ill. In the first place, it is essentially a passive system, that is, it does not go into operation until a patient takes the initiative by visiting a physician or a clinic. Often by the time a patient with a chronic illness takes this step it is late in the progress of the disease. For many of the chronic diseases much of the treatment is directed to symptoms rather than being curative. The regime of treatment is also likely to be protracted and costly. Another type of problem is that the system is geared to the one-to-one, episodic relationship in which the patient sees a physician, receives treatment and pays a fee. The system is unwieldy and inefficient when, as is often the case with chronic disease, the patient requires care by several physicians with different specialties, by other professional people such as nurse, therapists and social workers and by different institutions. Finally, the system is in a better position to take care of the patient who is incapacitated that he has to be in the hospital bed than the patient who is ill but more or less able to go about his normal business—and such patients constitute about 85 percent of the total. (pp. 14–15)

Chronic conditions, in particular, diabetes, arthritis, hypertension, and kidney disease, account for the rise in Medicare spending for the 20-year period from 1987 to 2006. The major factors that explain this growth in Medicare expenditures relate to more treatment of these diseases, in outpatient settings, and the common wisdom among physicians to start treating these conditions earlier than in the past, particularly hypertension. Thorpe, Ogden, and Galactionova 2010) found that

> The top-ten medical conditions accounted for approximately half of the inflation-adjusted rise in Medicare spending over the two decade period—47 percent from 1987 to 1997 and 51 percent from 1997 to 2006. (p. 719)

With many of Medicare-eligible individuals living with multiple chronic illnesses, the health care delivery system and its financing seems geared to an earlier age of episodic intervention to deliver acute care, mainly in hospital settings. Aligning the finances of care with the services required seems to be out of the picture. The transition to community care will require a whole new way of thinking about how to pay for it, especially for those individuals still covered by employer-based insurance and first-dollar responsibility going to the employee.

Some of the recent cost shifting in health insurance coverage to keep premiums down has impacted people with chronic illnesses. Paez, Zhao, and Hwang (2009) point out that the restructuring of payments for care under employer-sponsored health insurance plans allocate more of the financial burden to beneficiaries than in the past. The hand-off to beneficiaries of charges for medical care is not so much in the form of shared responsibility for premiums but the addition of copays and deductibles, particularly onerous charges for users of services who may need treatment or be followed by doctors and meaningless for the nonusers. Copayments and deductibles are designed to get consumers to pay attention to health care costs since they now have some "skin in the game" when it comes to deciding, "Shall I go to the doctor or wait and see if I feel better tomorrow?" This approach has some promise and it may all be to the good when you are dealing with the "worried well." However, there are special costs borne by those who are the sickest and once identified with a serious chronic illness, the costs start to escalate. Consider people with one, two, or three chronic illnesses that need interventions, usually in the form of medical visits or nursing care; they will be paying considerably more out-of-pocket for their medical care than their fellow workers who have no chronic conditions. Staying well may mean lower out-of-pocket expenses but it also means that the social compact side of insurance is ignored to save money for the employer who furnishes health plans to employees and their families.

How medical services are paid for through insurance plans can make a difference in the utilization of services for people still in the national workforce. In fact, based on conversations where people take me into their confidence, I surmise that people in the workforce don't want to mention that they get sick, lest the information get back to their employers. Even when much of the cost comes out-of-pocket, rather than being reimbursed by insurance, there is still reluctance to appear to be costly to employers. Moreover, chronic illness may keep people in the workforce when they are under 65 years of age, just so they can retain their medical benefits. Those with good benefits and a reason to use them may also be reluctant to relocate to a better job, lest the benefit package be less than what they are getting.

Individually purchased policies are exceptionally expensive, compared to the experience-rated group policies available through employment, where premiums are shared between employers and employees. Moreover, group sales by insurance companies are far more efficient in terms of cost effectiveness than seeking to sell to an individual. In addition, a person with a serious chronic illness will have a difficult time getting underwriting from a private insurance company. These commercial enterprises get to be financial giants not by efficiencies but by avoiding risk; the biggest risks are beneficiaries that actually will make claims. Turning down a person with a preexisting condition is done by all companies that sell individual policies. Getting access to a policy, despite preexisting conditions, with guaranteed issue, is likely to come about through health care reform since the Patient Protection and Affordable Care Act (PPACA) calls for elimination of those restrictions on sales. The insurance industry agreed to this as a tradeoff for the opportunity to sell policies through an insurance exchange to the millions of Americans, mostly the young and healthy, who will be required to buy coverage on their own. The individual mandate also makes sense from the perspective of the need to create an insurance pool that includes the healthy, whether temporarily or permanently so, and those with conditions that need attention.

I note that we might find some shifts in the labor force as a result of access to affordable coverage via the Affordable Care Act, the short name for PPACA. There are women in late middle age who work in low-paying clerical and secretarial jobs, as well as sales associate positions, to get coverage for themselves and their spouses through a group policy. The opportunity to access subsidies for health insurance policy purchases, or a lowering of premiums via the competition generated by the insurance exchange, where policies can be compared according to coverage and costs, may lead to early retirements. In addition, people who have been rejected for preexisting conditions by insurers or employers who want to keep their premiums down when purchasing experience rated group policies may be able to buy reasonably priced policies on their own. Consequently, we can ponder the intriguing question of how many marriages are kept together to manage the extremely high cost of health insurance in the United States.

Nevertheless, the problem of chronic disease will not go away so long as there are writers (DeVol and Bedroussian, 2007) and think tanks, e.g., the Milken Institute, that will continue to focus on saving lives and increasing productivity and economic growth through prevention. For the Milken Institute, the goals stated in the previous sentence are a direct result of the declared war on obesity—the main reason Americans are unhealthy. While obesity is a weighty problem, it does not really present, as I will argue in this book, the magnitude of the problem.

Still, recent analysis based on the data derived from the Department of Agriculture's study of food insecurity in the United States suggests that the risk of going hungry promotes a preference for "energy-dense foods, increased body fat, and decreased lean muscle mass. Adults who anticipate future food scarcity also over-consume during periods when access to food is reliable. This overconsumption can contribute not only to the development of diabetes but also to poor glycemic control in people who already have diabetes" (Seligman and Schillinger, 2010, p. 6). I cannot help but note that too much of a good thing is great but it also can be dangerous for your health. Adults with an adequate budget for food can avoid hypoglycemia and multiple doctor visits while those with low income often engage in a balancing act wherein they "reduce the amount of medication they take in order to have enough money for food and conversely, going hungry in order to afford medications" (Seligman and Schillinger, 2010, p. 7).

The countries that are developing economically are also starting to imitate the patterns of illness and disability found in the United States. There is ample evidence that there is a global pandemic of chronic diseases, an observation that moved *Health Affairs* to devote several articles in the December 2010 issue to the disease burden found around the world. The Caribbean and Latin America are starting to show the patterns of disease found in the United States and Western Europe. Cardiovascular disease in 2004 accounted for 35 percent of all deaths in these regions, as compared to 10 percent for tuberculosis, HIV, and malaria combined. Type 2 diabetes has become widespread and lethal in Mexico, taking the lead as the number one cause of mortality among Mexican women and the second leading cause of death in men (Dentzer, 2010c, p. 2136). While Mexico gets a great deal of attention when the drug lords declare war on each other, sometimes spilling their feuds across the border with the United States, there are quieter problems that are not reported on the evening news. The alarm has been sounded by the Bill and Melinda Gates Foundation that the chronic disease spotlight is now shining on the Americas.

Reports from the Centers for Disease Control and Prevention, issued in 2010, suggest that obesity continues to rise in the United States at a shocking rate, with 2.4 million more people becoming obese between 2007 and 2009, contributing to a total of 72.5 million or 26.7 percent of the population (Grady, 2010, p. A11). This figure does not include those considered overweight but not obese. The findings in this report support the theories about food insecurity. Given easy access to processed foods and lack of physical activity, African Americans and Hispanics were disproportionately heavy compared to whites. Exercise is possible even if you don't join a health club or run 10 miles a day. In cities with more dependence on mass transit, the rates of obesity were lower than those that relied on cars for transportation. And the more education people attained, the less likely they were obese. These results were derived from a telephone survey, conducted in 2007, and there may be some underreporting of weight while over-reporting of height. The state of Colorado was singled out not just for having low rates of obesity but also for building bike and hiking trails to promote exercise. Moreover, the state, even prior to the construction of ways to promote physical activity, was noted for an outdoor culture, as indicated by my observation several years ago that the enormous ads in the Denver newspapers for the kinds of equipment that backpackers, climbers, and off-road bikers need reflected a positive attitude to the strenuous life. In fact, there is some anecdotal information that people relocate to Colorado so they can more easily pursue these interests in a backpack friendly environment.

Opportunity to be physically active needs to be supported by good nutrition. Learning how to manage one's weight needs to begin in elementary school. One of the ways we can do better in promoting a healthier society is to reduce serious barriers to maintaining an appropriate body mass according to height, to reduce food insecurity, and to create country-wide what President Franklin D. Roosevelt called "freedom from want."

Beyond making good nutrition available to all so that obesity can be reduced, there are non-behavioral factors that have made us an aging society. The structure of the insurance and payment system can alter behavior and that has consequences for an individual's health and well-being. When Medicare came into effect in 1965, for example, there was a rush for services since many who became eligible for that government administered program held off visiting the doctor or having an elective procedure done until they were covered. In 2005, the older the age cohort, the more likely that people will report that they have one or more chronic diseases. It is no surprise that 37 percent of the age group from 45 to 64 report no chronic diseases while only 13 percent of the age group from 65 to 79 report likewise. As expected, there are even fewer people in age brackets beyond 80 who report the absence of chronic illness. Disclosure may be prevented for those in the workforce by a fear, often well founded, that they could lose existing coverage, especially when needed, if the presence of a chronic illness was reported back to an employer or an insurer.

The definition of what constitutes the clinical presence of a disease has become defined downward over the years. At one time, among Medicare patients, people with disabilities were more likely to be treated for clinical conditions than people without disabilities (Thorpe and Howard, 2006). However, with the elderly living longer—and this trend continues to move upward—the rate of new disabilities in this population may decline but the numbers of people with disabilities may continue to increase because life expectancy increased. The same cannot be said about the incidence of chronic illnesses that continue to increase among the elderly. Reductions could occur through changes in behavior or lifestyle (e.g., more exercise and lower-fat diets) and partly due to the treatment of diseases earlier in life. Moreover, coordinated care, not yet available through Medicare, could make a huge difference in the quality of life, a real game changer when it comes to reducing mortality rates and health care costs. Currently, as noted by Thorpe (2009) in his testimony in the United States Senate in May 2009, "episodic, uncoordinated care is ineffective and inefficient for patients like most Medicare beneficiaries who have multiple, chronic morbidities" (p. 10).

Treatment styles are also subject to change, recently including introducing more aggressive medical involvement in the lives of patients. This may be illustrated by the increase in the number of knee replacements, largely done to help the well get around better. Between 1992 and 2000, spending per nondisabled Medicare beneficiary increased 82 percent, compared with 58 percent for those with one or two activities of daily living (ADL) limitations and 44 percent for those with five or more such limitations.

Much of the explanation for this intensification of treatment and the consequent increase in costs for Medicare was related to the prevalence of obesity, but more importantly, to the treatment of this population. "More than half of all beneficiaries report receiving medical treatment for five or more conditions during a year" (Thorpe and Howard, 2009, p. w185). With laboratory-derived definitions of disease or other kinds of measures (e.g., blood pressure) being defined downward, thereby lowering the bar to treatment, more and more Medicare patients are being treated and life expectancy is increasing.

While there are serious disparities in morbidity (rates of sickness) and mortality (death rates) within the U.S. population related to poverty and race, as noted in Chapter 1, and the United States still trails 14 other countries in life expectancy, the increase in life expectancy means that there are more older people around. In 2007, life expectancy at birth modestly rose 0.2 years to 77.9 years (Xu, Kochanek, and Tejada-Vera, 2009, p. 1). Declines in death from heart disease, stroke, diabetes, and cancer indicate that there are more people who need to address their chronic illnesses through lifestyle changes (exercise and diet) and starting and sticking with the regimen of daily doses of medication. Moreover, many of these individuals would be better served by receiving collaborative care that monitors their conditions while they remain in the community.

Thorpe acknowledged (2009, p. 6) that Medicare patients would benefit if the fee-for-service driven model, based on delivery of acute care, was replaced by the adoption of chronic care treatment models, with alternative payment systems. Other health policy experts, working from a population health perspective, recommend investments in health policies that support interventions that can promote better medical care management as well as prevention of disease (Kindig, Asada, and Booske, 2008, p. 2081). Decisions that establish cost-effective procedures, insofar as they encourage better medical care management, also extend lives and support a better quality of life.

The emphasis on rebasing medical care management and extending lives of good quality requires that patients are recognized as people and not as manageable commodities, something to be processed and moved on to the next stage of health care. This is particularly the plight of the elderly, who are receiving care often funded through Medicare. Rates of re-hospitalization for the formerly hospitalized within 30 days following discharge is established at 18 percent (Thorpe, 2009, p. 8). Often these costly and preventable readmissions are for elderly people. Given how lavishly we spend on health care annually, $7,290 per capita, compared to other countries, this kind of failure in treatment and discharge planning would seem to be unacceptable (Davis, Schoen, and Stremikis, 2010, p. 2).

So how can delivery system practices be improved? There are numerous models to choose from. For the elderly, doctors such as Dennis McCullough, a family physician in New Hampshire, advocate that patients receive family centered care that avoids exhausting diagnostic tests and complex medication regimens. He calls for the development of an advocacy team of friends and relatives who constitute a "circle of concern" and protection (Zuger, 2008). Standard medical care often does not include family and friends and is fragmented so that there is no physician or other health-care provider acting as the care coordinator for the patient. Called "slow medicine," this fad is emulating the popular "slow food" movement. It is based on the idea that protecting the hospitalized and/or the discharged patient requires humanistic approaches that can go beyond sophisticated medical care. The suggestion is not that less is more but that a different strategy is required to get people discharged from hospitals and into their homes. The circle of concern approach has been adopted by state agencies attempting to return people with intellectual and developmental disabilities back into the community. The members of the circle are especially critical to coordination at times of changes in the care team.

The transition point—when a person with a chronic illness leaves one set of providers—is a moment for communication to break down. Smother, safer, and more effective "hand offs" are extremely important for helping patients manage in the community. The United Hospital Fund's Next Step in Care is an attempt, according to spokesperson David A. Gould, "to change health care practice so that family caregivers are routinely included in transition planning and implementation, and we want to improve family caregivers' knowledge and skills so that they can be more effective partners" (Blueprint, 2009, p. 1).

There is another meaning of transition in medical settings and an issue raised, aside from going from the hospital bed to return home to the one's home and family caregivers—a concern based on the way in which medicine is organized. Sometimes the hand-off to other providers cannot take place because there is no one out there answering the request for age-appropriate help. Children with chronic illnesses may receive extended services from pediatricians for their primary care far beyond children who do not have these conditions. Disease-specific voluntary associations have often sought out medical professionals to help address this problem so that there will be a seamless transition for adolescents to adult medical care for individuals with such conditions as spina bifida, asthma, and hemophilia. With data collected in 2005–2006 from the National Survey of Children with Special Health Care Needs, the Health Resources and Services Administration (HRSA, 2010) found that nationally close to 17 percent of adolescents between the ages of 12 and 17 had either a serious chronic illness or a disability. For this vulnerable population, nearly one out of five teenagers, how the switch is made is important for health maintenance.

While readers may anticipate that there are serious problems in transition for young adults, Scal (2002) surprisingly found that "two large population-based studies suggest that many young adults with chronic conditions appear to make the transition into adulthood without serious ill effects" (p. 1315). Yet young adults, parents, and physicians, especially pediatricians, found that the most serious problem in transition was identifying adult primary care providers. Providers who were nominated by various disease-oriented voluntary associations were most concerned about having enough skill and time to devote to individualizing the service needs of adult patients with childhood acquired chronic illnesses. This kind of customizing of care would involve not only addressing the medical needs introduced by a chronic condition but also present and anticipated changes in behavior, sexuality, and reproduction (Scal, 2002, p. 1319).

Transition may also mean recognition that one is now a member of a community of others who are similarly situated, e.g., a person with lupus. In sum, we cannot comment on chronic illness without addressing the human side—what it means existentially and identity wise to be chronically ill. The national media, in following people with chronic illnesses, raise the question of whether they act just like everyone else. The discovery is that reporters and survey researchers note that they are less likely to use or have access to the Internet than people without these lifelong conditions. However, a disproportionate share of people with chronic illnesses are poorer, older, or members of minority groups and thereby must overcome some financial and even social barriers to become part of a cyberspace nation. This is especially true of people managing multiple illnesses. But there is something significant to report how chronic illness may limit interest in the Internet as a way of securing information and communicating with others with the same disease or on a multi-disease blog:

when all of these demographic factors are controlled, living with a chronic illness in and of itself has an independent, negative effect on someone's likelihood to have internet access. (Fox and Purcell, 2010)

The Web does furnish the opportunity to become part of a virtual community made up of other people with similar needs for information and emotional support. The need for discussion and direction is just as important as it has always been when trying to get help for oneself or a loved one. Organizations such as New York City's Association for the Help of Retarded Children, the flagship chapter of the national network called Association for Retarded Citizens, was a haven in a heartless world in the 1960s and earlier for parents whose offspring were stigmatized and who themselves were shunned as a result. Today the plight of the chronically is discussed on the Internet.

> People fighting chronic illness are less likely than other to have internet access, but once online they are more likely to blog or participate in online discussions about health problems. (Miller, 2010)

Once on the Internet, people link rapidly to others who are similarly situated. Organizations on the World Wide Web have sprung up to reflect this new empowerment, with interesting names such as My Invisible Disabilities Community (invisibledisabilities.ning.com), Diabetic Connect (www.defeatdiabetes.com), and Patients Like Me (www.patientslikeme.com). No longer isolated because of the limits of access to people with the same condition when living in a small town, people in these networks swear by them. A 50-year-old man with multiple sclerosis and recovering from brain cancer said, "It really literally saved my life, just to be able to connect with other people" (Miller, 2010).

Being in the same boat gives diabetics, for example, a chance to develop realistic perspectives on the disease via an opportunity to talk with others experiencing the same physical and psychosocial sensations. These networks are now part of the health care delivery system, whether providers are comfortable with their patients using them or not, just in the same way that patients use complementary and alternative medicine (CAM) along with the Western and scientific variety, because it gives them a sense of control over their own lives. Perhaps this energized part of the chronic illness population can give a shout out to the more electronically isolated and talk to them. Moreover, there is a need for them to be active in taking advantage of the more engaging nature of health care institutions as they now welcome participation from their consumers and so learn how to make care better

(Foubister, 2010). Participation in advisory councils might be difficult for some people with chronic illnesses but they can supply some incredible insights into how the health care delivery system works or fails to deliver what is promised.

The Internet is no longer the luxury it once was and people with chronic illnesses should get linked up. Consider the possibility of the government issuing a laptop with Web access, often inexpensively accessible via land telephone lines, or even better, the family contributing to the purchase of the laptop to the person who is isolated and electronically challenged. How different is this communication linkage from the availability of funds for transportation for some Medicaid eligible individuals so they can get to their medical appointments?

## WHY DELIVERY SYSTEM REFORM?

While it is often said in the field of communications that less is more, there are also some excellent reasons to say "Whoa!" when it comes to medical care. Yes, there is a concern expressed among health care system experts that too much medical care can be exhausting, especially for the frail elderly person. Conversely, there is substantial quantifiable evidence that perhaps the Medicare-covered population get too little of the medical care they need. As mentioned by Thorpe (2009, p. 2)—and this comes as a bit of a shock—more than half of all Medicare beneficiaries are treated annually for five of more chronic conditions. Another way of slicing the data and demonstrating the impact on the health care price tag nationally is that nine conditions account for 60 percent of the rise of Medicare spending in the last decade. Most of the recommended care required is not in hospitals but is in the patient's home. If these patients receive the recommended care, then patients are more likely to be stabilized and are apt to, more or less, pick up their lives where they left them before the onset of a downturn in their health. Strikingly, there is evidence to show that 45 percent of patients do not get clinically recommended services. There are a number of factors that promote the failure to receive these vital services.

There are often limited kinds of planning prior to the patient's discharge. Concern about getting the patient out and about and the bed reoccupied may leave hospital administrators and medical staff uninterested in looking at how badly they are performing in this area of care and unwilling to go the extra mile to make the transition seamless. Real effort to bridge the gap may pay off in reduced readmissions. Robust patient discharge planning can make for a reversal, or improvement, of the odds that a patient will be readmitted. The process has to involve real service delivery, including as Amy Boutwell (2010) at the Institute for Healthcare Improvement suggests, "engaging patients or their families or caregivers as partners in care, using anticipatory guidance for self-care needs, appropriately mobilizing support and follow-up, and communicating directly and promptly with the receiving clinicians" (p. 1244). In other words, how the care is delivered is just as important as the medical content.

One great structural limitation to furnishing coordinated care to newly discharged patients is the limited size of primary care provider practices in the United States, with one or two provider practices still found to be the modal type. Overcoming this limitation to coordination requires the building of community-wide care coordination units that can become partners with the solo practitioner or with those in two or three primary care provider (PCP) groups. These practices often have few options when it comes to delegating tasks and so the more resources are brought in from the outside, the more effective and efficient community care will be.

A second great structural limitation is related to the Medicare fee-for-service payment system, one in which most beneficiaries are enrolled. Although the Medicare Advantage programs are evidently overpaid for the services provided and subject to correction via PPACA, they do permit funding for care coordination in a far less restrictive way than in fee-for-service Medicare. Health care reform legislation, once passed, will make it possible to pay for Medicare services in a bundled fashion, thereby allowing for care coordinators to be funded. Management of chronic illness both inside the hospital and outside would require the creation of primary care delivery teams that would receive the bundled payments (Luft, 2009, p. 625). There is no way to support these teams via a fee-for-service approach. Still, caution is required when dealing with a population that can destabilize.

Making this new payment system—the bundled payment arrangement—work is not going to be easy. One size may not fit all. Experts such as Berenson and Rich (2010) point out that the bundled payment system is fraught with dangers when dealing with patients with high levels of acuity, brought on by various circumstances, including having to deal with patients with several chronic illnesses who are presenting with acute problems. Few primary care physicians are trained to deliver this kind of care and would want to take on these kinds of patients unless well compensated.

Even caring for acute, minor illnesses varies depending on the presence of co-morbidities. While many of these chronic illnesses cluster together, e.g., hypertension, congestive heart failure, diabetes, chronic renal failure, etc., current episode payment approaches (as well as clinical practice guidelines and Pay for Performance measures) generally assume independence of these conditions. Indeed, even the concept of an episode of a chronic condition might be viewed as an oxymoron since they generally do not end, except in death. (p. 617)

Third, hospitals are not incentivized to avoid readmissions. Like a bank considered too big to fail, the contemporary hospital administration does not lose anything when a patient is readmitted. Another way of putting it is that there are no risks for the hospital if the patient returns. In fact, readmission keeps up the demand for hospital beds and therefore is a way of rewarding poor decision making in the patient discharge planning phase. Called "frequent flyers" by the overworked house staff (now all designated as residents) of medical centers, there are some patients who move in and out of the hospital at high rates. Reductions in the rate of hospitalization and the average length of stay will help bend the cost curve in health care in the United States as well as encourage more independence on the part of people with chronic illnesses.

The Affordable Care Act will fund bundled payment demonstrations through Section 3022 in the year 2013, after establishing the guidance for these programs. Clearly, these efforts are supportive of patient-centered medical homes and accountable care organizations. The argument so far is that there are cost savings generated in Center for Medicare and Medicaid Services funded (Cromwell et al., 1998) and provider-sponsored projects (Casale et al., 2007) ranging from 5 to 10 percent.

Based on a specific mandate from Congress in 2000, the Department of Health and Human Services was directed to promote care coordination, increase efficiency, and incentivize doctors to promote better health outcomes. Medicare's Physician Group Practice Demonstration continued to pay doctors on a fee-for-service basis but also offered performance payments via an 80 percent share of the savings accrued to Medicare. Rewards were based specifically on meeting quality and cost targets, with groups generating a "Medicare savings of $38.7 million, earning performance payments of $31.7 million" (Iglehart, 2010b, p. 2). It should be noted that where there were participating hospitals, the demonstration did not produce savings and there were no financial penalties for failing to hit the targets.

Any efforts to establish bundled payment methods require that there be strong ties between hospitals and providers in the community. Given the history of competition, cooperation is not something to be taken for granted. One way that cooperation can be increased is through developing coordinated information systems that allow for easy sharing of patient data and financial histories. Information systems will also have to include new systems of billing that are compatible with basing payment on episodes of treatment and care.

There are some pilot programs that are community minded and consumer minded at the same time. The idea is to create a delivery system that encourages more self-management, making it possible for chronic disease care to make the patient a partner in his or her own support. This does not mean that people with a chronic disease are simply trained and left to sink or swim on their own. Rather, there is an effort to create a support system with the help of nonphysician staff such as licensed vocational nurses or community health workers. The nature of these diseases cries out for this kind of intervention.

Susan Baird Kanaan (2008) reported on the lessons learned through an initiative to support self-management for patients with diabetes, an expensive disease and one where diabetics can learn various self-management techniques. Ten health care organizations around the state of California participated in this pilot project, one where the delivery system became more user-friendly, where support staff were exposed to a long one-day training session, conducted by a diabetes expert, and where the impact of program participation was measured at all sites. Close analysis of each location via case studies revealed some important insights into the value of this program. At one health maintenance organization (HMO), patients found in group discussion that there was strong value in follow-up phone calls to help them stay concentrated on their action plans and focused on tracking medications and laboratory tests (Kanaan, 2008, p. 14). At another location, the provider team was enthusiastic and felt they could extend the self-management model to care for people with other chronic conditions such as asthma and hypertension.

Beyond the confines or freedoms of self-management, other innovators have found that the interest in family involvement in chronic care has been driven by the idea that much can be done in the community with the help of a support team that is part of patient-centered primary care. When family members feel close to each other, this foundation helps providers involve everyone in the household and others within traveling distance into patient self-management.

As one might anticipate, a good deal of the training of family members to assist people with chronic illnesses involves the acquisition of communications skills. Clearly, a person who wants to help may also be obstructive if the message is presented in a way that does not support the patient's sense of well-being—e.g., the family caregiver who acts in a controlling fashion ("you know that you can't eat candy") or assumes they are in charge now that a loved one has a chronic illness ("I always take him to Joey's restaurant because I can get him a simple meal, without fats"). There are better ways of expressing concern without belittling the person.

Ann-Marie Rosland (2009), a physician at the Ann Arbor (Michigan) Healthcare System, has reported "background information, experience-based insights, case examples, and further resources" for an audience of practitioners interested in extending family involvement in chronic care management (p. 2). Her observations supplied interesting contrasts between good communication among family members and poor communication, why it is different in caring for a person with a minor disability and one with an advanced disability, and how to do couples-oriented education focusing on the major topics involved in self-help and where the other member of a couple can furnish genuine assistance.

Nevertheless, there is a kind of silo effect in the U.S. world of health care, where the personal constraints of having to cope with a chronic illness are discussed in terms of the consequences for the professional, since personal identity is sometimes questioned and primary group relationships (e.g., family and domestic partnerships) are often strained (Buckley, 2008). While doctors may be taught to learn how to talk to patients about sensitive issues, there is no indication that these communication skills might also help patients take advantage of some new concepts in chronic care management—the patient-centered medical home.

The Affordable Care Act has some funding for institution building of the kind that will promote greater care coordination, particularly of the kind that generates savings to Medicare as well as create valuable community resources. Karen Davis (2010), the executive director of the Commonwealth Fund, in writing in the fund's blog summarizes some of the essentials the Affordable Care Act will put in place for moving forward.

> Moreover, the law creates a Center for Medicare and Medicaid Innovation to pilot new ways of paying for and delivering health care, including "bundled" methods of payment to encourage providers to work together across health care settings to treat their patients and approaches that reward those who offer appropriate, high-quality, and efficient care. (p. 1)

While payment structures matter, there is also much to overcome in the culture of health care to make these changes happen. Professions can be well defended when it comes to responding to innovations, even those who gain in importance through the introduction of care coordination. In a collection of essays on chronic illness, a kind of reader for students, focusing on its impact and interventions and aimed at the nursing profession, the authors surprisingly make no mention of new models of chronic care. Lubkin and Larsen (2006) edited an anthology, now in its sixth edition, that breaks down how the patient with a chronic illness presents various challenges to nursing staff. It is a list of what to watch out for—from social roles assumed to the physical stresses experienced—without any holistic effort to demonstrate how primary care, built around patient involvement and self-management within the context of a physician-led multidisciplinary team, can be adapted to the demands and expectations associated with serious chronic illness. This is a glaring omission in a text for new members of the profession of nursing, a profession that will play a key and critical role in improving chronic care coordination.

Even the editors of the *New York Times* (2010a), in seeking to point out how the cost of health care increases the deficit, fail to mention the new partnerships between consumers and providers of health care, but rather focus singly on the hard-wired system innovations that the Affordable Care Act will permit.

> **Fixing the System** The best way to lower health care spending is to reform the dysfunctional health care system whose costs seem unrelated to the quality of care delivered. The reform law makes a good start, sponsoring research to determine which treatments are effective and which are not, starting pilot projects to change the way care is delivered and paid for, and setting up new organizations to rush successful approaches into wide use in Medicare and ultimately the private sector. (p. wk 7)

Both the emphasis on self-management and the role of the family are relatively new approaches to the problem of chronic care in the community; the development of interest in these topics is fueled by the widely held view by health delivery system experts and health policy analysts that the U.S. approach to chronic care is broken and needs to be rebuilt. In the next chapter, I will examine the current system that is in place for delivery of services to people with chronic illnesses and the extent to which it is aligned or misaligned with the problem.

# 3

# How Well Does U.S. Medicine Deal with Chronic Illness?

U.S. medicine is built on a payment structure and a technology that rewards the treatment of acute conditions. The surgeon who is given, for example, an acute appendicitis to cure via the removal of that vestigial organ has at his or her disposal a decisive technological intervention. The surgeon and his or her team can usually eliminate the pain and potential sepsis for the patient through action while the patient merely has to give consent. Generally, the surgeon is pleased to get a referral and is paid itemized fees for the services rendered. There may not be an inconvenient time to go to work when one is paid on what can be considered piecework. A salaried surgeon, in contrast, might not mind doing the work involved but could be unhappy about being taken off the tennis court or from a daughter's field hockey match to help a patient in urgent need.

The way that U.S. doctors think about their work according to those who seek systemic change, such as CEO Mark D. Smith of the California Healthcare Foundation, is also being called into question. Getting physicians to pay attention to population characteristics is a major challenge, according to Smith.

> The way I was trained and the way most docs practice, that's not the deal—the deal is, you see patients one at a time as they come in. Yet it's very clear that we can't improve the care of people with chronic diseases unless we get providers starting to think about the population of people with diseases. Most docs, even doctors in multispecialty practices or in groups, haven't organized their practices that way. So registries of similar groups of patients have to be the underpinning to help providers understand what their outcomes are with groups of patients over time. (Dentzer, 2010, p. 295)

In nations similar to the United States with regard to economic development, there may be standard prices set for procedures that are arrived at by a government commission. In some countries, the price for a physician's service is set via negotiation by the national government and the national medical society. Where health insurance is supplied by a private corporation, there usually are restrictions on making profits on health insurance, thereby making it possible to offer coverage at a lower price. Private insurers are allowed to make profits on insurance for other items, such as access to a private room. In addition, everyone must have insurance coverage, which brings into the risk pool many able-bodied people who will not seek a great deal of health care but will have their care paid for if they do require care. The mutuality of the system makes it financially sustainable.

Receiving an appendectomy also involves hospitalization. The patient who is hospitalized for this procedure usually is insured and payment is made on the basis of prospective formula, i.e., what the average length of stay is for this diagnostic related treatment. These treatments, for simplicity's sake, are grouped according to the organ system involved and as a payment system was initially introduced as a formula for hospitals in the 1980s for Medicare beneficiaries. The diagnostic related groups (DRG) or prospective payment system was widely adopted by private insurers and helped to greatly reduce the costs of hospital care.

However, for one out of five patients, DRGs have promoted the use of a revolving door. The facts show that there have been numerous hospitalizations following the initial discharge within the U.S. hospital system. As noted in the last chapter, the national average is around 18 percent in the first 30 days following discharge and is considered by health care services experts to be largely unnecessary and extremely costly. Rehospitalization leads to a new round of payments for doctors and hospitals because the fee-for-service system and the DRGs, in contrast to a bundled payment system, allow for additional charges, usually welcomed by the health care providers.

Many rehospitalizations and additional treatments for avoidable relapses are considered by experts a result of the underdevelopment of chronic care services in the United States. As Ken Thorpe and Lydia Ogden concluded in 2009, "Episodic, uncoordinated care is ineffective and inefficient for patients like most Medicare beneficiaries who have multiple chronic co-morbidities" (p. 5). While patients may not be capable of articulating this summary statement, the data back up what Thorpe and Ogden suggest are the reasons for rehospitalization. It is evident that the coordination of care is not well supported by Medicare's fee structure. Medicare beneficiaries who are discharged from hospitals and admitted to skilled nursing facilities for post-acute care have a one in four chance of being readmitted to the hospital within 30 days (Mor, Intrator, Feng, and Grabowski, 2010, p. 57). In fact, it may be financially advantageous to the hospital and the skilled nursing facility for patients to be moving back and forth since the hospital gets paid on a per diem basis and the skilled nursing facility, often paid on a flat rate by the state Medicaid system, may have a bed freed up to be used while the patient is in the hospital. The estimated cost to Medicare was $4.34 billion in 2006. The impact on the elderly patient who is shuttled back and forth can be physically stressful and devastating emotionally; furthermore, hospital care also increases the likelihood of medical errors when there is a failure of care coordination.

Hospital stays might be reasonable ways to assist patients in their return to the activities they enjoyed before being admitted. However, there is no reason to treat a hospital stay as always to the benefit of the patient. A hospital stay can be dangerous to your health! Four years after the Institute of Medicine's (IOM) report about the many medical mistakes that seriously affected the health of patients, a recent study of the period 2002 to 2007 of North Carolina hospitals found that some of the most frequently identified problems could have been avoided, particularly if patients were not spending so many days as inpatients. Hospital acquired infections, adverse drug affects, and falls would not have been such common occurrences if patients were discharged sooner (Landrigan et al., 2010). The IOM's report did launch many efforts to correct conditions that resulted in patient harm, but little change was demonstrated in the rates of error in the 10 hospitals reviewed.

Care coordination may also be justified following hospitalization by the fact that for some older Americans who were treated in hospitals for critical illnesses, or even noncritical illnesses, hospitalization promotes the onset of dementia. Ehlenbach and his colleagues (2010) sought "to determine whether decline in cognitive function was greater among older individuals who experience acute care or critical illness hospitalizations relative to those not hospitalized and to determine whether the risk for incident dementia differed by these exposures" (p. 763). They found that the odds were greater that those hospitalized, either for critical or noncritical illnesses, compared to those who remained in the community, would develop dementia. Care coordination can do much of the heavy lifting to help those discharged to minimize the impact of dementia.

## DESPERATE CORPORATIONS

The cost of the failure of care coordination is also borne by employers who, in response to this burden, have created their own version of the medical home to reduce their expenditures on chronic care and keep valued employees from missing work. The range of services found at the workplace can vary from a simple reminder call to a employee to take a medication or get a test done in a timely fashion to the use of nurses with special training to work directly with a patient to make sure that he or she is stable, receives the right medication, and makes adjustments in diet and other aspects of the way he or she lives (Konrad, 2010, p. B6).

Feedback from employees suggests that they have learned to appreciate the extra help. A Boeing engineer was better able to manage his chronic pulmonary problem with the help of a few reminders, courtesy of one of the major aircraft manufacturers on the planet.

> That prompting allowed me to think a little bit more carefully about a nagging problem I was putting off or that I might not have remembered to mention at an annual check-up. She can go and talk to any of my doctors, get me an answer or tell me who I should go see. (qtd. in Konrad, 2010, p. B6)

The issue of care coordination can be significant if there is no communication between the nurse at the factory or office and the primary care physician. Bringing the primary care doctor into the picture means letting him or her know about prescriptions authorized by company doctors at no or little cost to encourage patient compliance. It is important to complete the circle so there are no adverse drug interactions or duplications of medicines.

Companies such as Boeing, Pitney Bowes, and Quad/Graphics, a Wisconsin-based printing company, have had good results when it comes to improved productivity and lower costs from 20 to 30 percent per enrollee in the chronic care programs (Konrad, 2010, p. B6). And since these companies are self-insured, the savings are direct. Yet there may come a time when coordinated care is affordable and available and companies will no longer need to support workplace nursing.

The emphasis on corporations reaching employees as a show of concern for wellness has been picked up by the Center for Studying Health System Change and is considered a way to transform primary care. In a detailed qualitative policy paper (Ha, Boukus, and Cohen, 2010) the center presents clinical management models, types of clinical services (including disease management), and several clinic primary care delivery models. The paper suggests that "In the long run, improving population health by preventing and managing chronic conditions is a major objective" (p. 2). Furthermore, the authors also identify employee financial incentives for clinic use, staffing and recruiting, startup challenges, as well as the governmental environment and whether dependents can utilize these clinics.

An older worker with one or more chronic conditions may find it better to stop working and seek eligibility for federal disability payments derived from an insurance program created by Congress in 1956. Access to benefits not only means that the applicant is deemed unable to be fully employable but is also entitled to receive Medicare benefits prior to the retirement age of 65. While the number of applicants for these monthly benefits and health insurance has increased substantially during the last four years, according to Peter Orszag (2010, p. A35), the former director of the White House Office of Management and Budget, there is good reason to consider that some of the pressure for eligibility is related to the increasing number of people in the workforce with several chronic illnesses. Some of them can be assisted by reorganization of the health care delivery system that fails to deliver appropriate chronic care at reasonable cost to people who could remain employed if they received it. Alternatively, without these supports, individual workers who are on the border of eligibility for Supplemental Security Disability Income may seek it not just because it is there but because working has become too physically challenging.

## ENCOURAGEMENT VIA THE AFFORDABLE CARE ACT

At this point in time, these corporate-based programs can be models for what needs to be done. Given the patient need and the built-in waste in the system, it is urgent for health planners to scale up the delivery of chronic care. With invasive treatments of patients with chronic illnesses and their subsequent care fueling 75 percent of health care spending, it is extremely important to make this care more effective and more efficient. There is a disconnect between what patients with chronic illnesses should receive and what they actually get. As mentioned in the previous chapter, it is estimated that patients with chronic illnesses only receive a little more than half of the clinically recommended services (Thorpe and Ogden, 2009, p. 1), hardly the gold standard for care. Therefore, patients often are not able to escape from avoidable complications following medical or surgical treatment.

There is also the point in chronic care where, near the end of life, patients get too much in the way of technological interventions and too little in the way of "avoiding suffering, being with family, having the touch of others, being mentally aware, and not becoming a burden to others," all concerns expressed in surveys by patients with terminal illness (Gawande, 2010, p. 39). For many people with various comorbidities acquired during old age, it is extremely difficult to know when to resist these major but mostly indecisive interventions and live out the remainder of one's life with hope but with some pleasure and even joy.

Remaking chronic care could also take these concerns about the end of life, as expressed by terminally ill people, into account in establishing coordinated care teams and designing how to work with patients when they destabilized. Some students of chronic care delivery are surely aware of this need. The improvement of chronic care could also be a major way to "reduce duplication of services, reduce administrative waste, and improve outcomes" (Weinstein and Skinner, 2010, p. 463), a way to eliminate unnecessary services. Money spent wisely on these services can make a big difference in improving "functional status, quality of life, disability, major clinical events, and death" (Neumann and Tunis, 2010, p. 377).

Patients eligible for Medicaid are disproportionately likely to have chronic illnesses and disabilities. The 2010 Patient Protection and Affordable Care Act (PPACA), as if on cue, created a state option to provide health homes for Medicaid enrollees with chronic conditions. There is $25 million available through the Secretary of Health and Human Services to support planning of "health homes" furnished by a designated provider, including many different health professionals and organizations. Section 2703 of PPACA stipulates that the entity that receives the grant must provide "comprehensive case management, care coordination and health promotion, transitional care, patient and family support, referral to community services, and the use of health information technology, as appropriate" (Pulse, 2010, p. 14).

With these incentives and certification standards come analytic and reporting responsibilities. The states that receive funds to develop medical homes for Medicaid beneficiaries who qualify for coordinated chronic care will also be required to do independent evaluations, to be completed by January 2017. The states will also furnish interim information on the steps they took to create coordinated care and lessons learned (Bernstein, Chollet, Peikes, and Peterson, 2010, p. 4).

With regard to Medicare, the Affordable Care Act, as PPACA has become known, will allow the Center on Medicare and Medicaid Services (CMS) to go beyond pilot and demonstration projects, encouraging group practices, independent practice associations, networks of practitioners, collaborations of hospitals, and other groups that employ professionals to participate as accountable care organizations (ACOs), or provider partnerships that are quality oriented, patient centered, and driven by incentives to reduce overall spending growth for defined populations. According to a 2010 Health Policy Brief, jointly written by *Health Affairs* and the Robert Wood Johnson Foundation,

> Each ACO must have a formal legal structure that will allow it to receive shared savings payments and distribute them among providers, and it must show that it can meet quality and reporting standards to be developed by the secretary (of HHS). (Merlis, 2010, p. 5)

The Affordable Care Act not only seeks savings but will require performance measurement of providers to make sure that they are doing better or as well by their patients as providers who are not linked through a ACO structure or who are not assigned to the ACO but see the same providers.

Beyond quality issues, questions have been raised such as the following:

- Can providers realize the same incomes when they reduce service to affect savings when they are no longer working in a fee-for-service payment system?
- What happens to projected savings if providers who have a large volume of patients and create highly integrated systems may also be in a better bargaining position with insurance companies and managed care plans and therefore drive up costs?
- Are the start-up incentives sufficient to encourage scaled-up participation when there are substantial front-end costs that these new ACOs will have to bear, including investments in electronic medical record systems (Merlis, 2010, p. 4)?

## CHRONIC CARE: MEDICINE'S ORPHAN

Why is chronic care so ineffective? The full story of chronic care in the United States has to be understood as an undeveloped territory of medicine, a new frontier in most parts of the country. The programs that get it right are pilot projects or integrated health systems such as Kaiser that receive little attention from consumers but are often highlighted in efforts to convince the public that health care reform is possible and has real care benefits as well as being important. Health care spending cannot be reduced without better targeted services so that patients are kept from declining physically and thereby becoming good candidates for hospital admissions.

Most provider practices in the United States, as mentioned in Chapter 2, owing to their size, are not set up to generate a plan and team for a patient in the community who needs chronic care. It is no wonder that Americans with chronic illnesses, compared to adults from seven other equally developed countries, are far more likely to report that they had access problems due to cost (54%), coordination problems such as a failure to receive test results at the time of appointments (34%), and medical, medication, or laboratory errors (34%). These negative experiences go counter to the claims often made by supporters of the status quo in health care that we already are blessed by a high-performance health care system and no reforms of the delivery system are required (Voelker, 2008). The cheerleading for the current health care system is spearheaded by people who never met a corporation that they didn't like and who espouse a kind of bright-sided populism that regards the small business owner at the backbone of our civilization. They deeply resent large twenty-first-century multinational corporations, staffed by well-educated individuals who were not from small towns in rural America or were not even born in the United States. These populists, found in the Tea Party, have uncovered a raw nerve of resentment that is based on the belief that people are being processed in the name of a medical science establishment that has no interest in letting them have control over their own lives. Paradoxically, right-wing populists have ridden the alienation theme of 1960s' radicals, stealing their passion, but mostly to smother concern about creating more equality via government intervention.

And there is some merit in their argument, a truth first recognized by Students for a Democratic Society and other New Left groups in the 1960s when their young leaders sought to speak truth to power. There are defenders of our health care system who say that the medical humanism movement—an effort to understand the individual's cultural preferences, values, and objectives in seeking care—is an important asset in what can be a highly impersonal world. This kind of approach goes beyond guidance and cooperation, the way a physician may instruct diabetic patients on how to monitor their condition to make sure that they have correct blood sugar levels. The goal of humanistic medicine is to make treatment a mutually participatory experience for provider and patient. This kind of approach is best exemplified by psychotherapy but it also is the foundation of how doctors and patients negotiate end-of-life care, with the patient essentially stating what kinds of invasive procedures he or she will tolerate and which ones he or she will not (Hartzband and Groopman, 2009, p. 1350). Moreover, it is the humanistic approach to medical care that allows patients to determine under what conditions they want to be kept alive when suffering from a terminal illness such as pancreatic cancer. Moreover, as cures develop or, more likely, as drugs and other interventions are found to extend life, then these discussions regarding a specific illness may be unnecessary and a disease gets dropped from the non-curable list.

Mutual participation is extremely appropriate for dealing with patients with multiple problems and where formula cannot be followed. Considering how many older Americans have several chronic diseases at the same time, it is also important to note that the array of coexisting morbidities often makes the use of clinical practice guidelines, or how-to-proceed manuals for doctors, difficult. A responsive provider can explain to a patient that the best care available, according to scientific results, may not be offered because of the complicated nature of the patient's various conditions. Still, consistency in the caregiving may help patients feel that they are being helped, even when the experts do not have a clear-cut treatment to follow. In sum, trust comes from the patient's perception that the doctor really cares.

There is growing evidence from international studies that plentiful primary care makes chronic care effective. Consistency in the form of continuity and comprehensiveness of care is the hallmark of the European and some Asian states, e.g., Taiwan, South Korea, most of which is based on a national health insurance model. Using the primary care provider to create the locus of care for patients is driven in these countries by the knowledge that this is both effective and less expensive than offering far more expensive and often unnecessary specialty care. In Denmark, for example, the entire health care system is organized around easily accessible primary care physicians, who establish patient-centered medical homes. This care system is buttressed by a sophisticated information system that enhances care coordination.

The Commonwealth Fund, a major policy-oriented foundation in this country, not only has the scoop on the Danish remodeling of their health care system but also found that in the United States, the management of chronic conditions for Medicare eligible patients improves significantly when the medical home is established, as noted in the Foundation's 2006 Medicare Chartbook.

Primary care has some serious backing from recent health care delivery system research. The esteemed Dartmouth Center for Evaluative Clinical Sciences in Hanover, New Hampshire, compared states that relied more on primary care with those that relied more on specialty care and found primary care permitted lower Medicare spending, lower resource utilization, including facilities and labor, lower utilization rates such as physician visits and days in the hospital, and better quality of care as measured by composite quality scores (Dartmouth Atlas of Health Care, 2006). Other health services research teams, such as the one headed by Barbara Starfield (Starfield et al., 2001), a distinguished Johns Hopkins faculty member, found lower resource utilization in domestic and foreign studies and lower mortality rates when adults with a primary care physician is in the picture as compared to specialty care.

T. R. Reid (2009), a U.S. journalist, brought the same complaint to primary care physicians in various countries in Europe and Asia to find out how they would differ in treating his declining shoulder injury, which reduced his range of motion significantly. He used this approach to write a charming book on the different health care systems he encountered on his way to getting medical attention. In some instances, the recommended course of treatment was physical therapy or even alternative healing. In most places the price of all treatments was publicly available. Most significantly, there was often an effort to make improvements in his physical condition without the use of high-tech surgery.

## MAKING COORDINATED CARE HAPPEN

The treatment of chronic illness requires the use of a care system that is coordinated so that all of the appropriate services are available and organized in such a way that the patient's condition does not worsen and may even improve as a result of interventions. This means that services that remain outside of the billing system are included and that the providers are held accountable for improved patient outcomes. Even with the expansion of coverage that is likely to occur via PPACA, just creating access to inferior practices or practitioners will not create the right kind of chronic care system (Commonwealth Fund Commission on a High Performance Health System, 2009). Primary care providers will have to be able not only to refer to subspecialists but also to treat chronic illnesses and manage coordinated care.

Mutual participation, hardly a new concept in describing doctor-patient relationships, may be the foundation of coordinated care. The California Health Care Foundation (CHCF)—built on Blue Cross of California's transfer of assets to the state so it could go for-profit—identified self-management support as a building block of chronic care that "transforms the patient-provider relationship into a collaborative partnership and organizes the health care team around the pivotal role of the patient" (Kanaan, 2008, p. 5). This new demonstration project was built on an earlier version called *Promoting Effective Self-Management Approaches to Improve Chronic Disease Care*, discussed in Chapter 2.

Committed to this approach, the CHCF in 2006 gave out 10 $65,000 awards to sustain two-year self-management support projects. Since the management of diabetes is of major concern to health care providers, patients were deemed in need to learn to follow diet and fitness or medication instructions. But before that could occur, a cadre of trainers had to learn how to do diabetes management. A behavioral trainer taught trainees who would then work with patients on how to be confident that the acquisition of self-management skills would produce the appropriate changes in behavior that can produce different and desired clinical outcomes.

The Chronic Care Model, upon which the self-management approaches are built, targets the health care system, the patient, and the provider. Patients and providers are brought into a partnership where they "identify health goals, choose specific actions, acquire needed information, and monitor progress" (Kanaan, 2008, p. 5). Through a question-and-answer approach, the self-directed patients come up with the right answers for how to achieve their goals. What information does the physician supply? Is it sound and based on scientific discovery of what works, and under what conditions, and what doesn't work, or in current parlance, evidence-based practice?

## EVIDENCE-BASED TREATMENT

We need to find answers to these questions because the U.S. health care system is expensive compared to what is spent in other countries (e.g., Great Britain, France, and Germany) and the results in the United States are less impressive. Chronic care requires a platform of well-tested treatments that are widely used by specialists with patients with similar kinds of illnesses.

Moreover, doctors have to use this information in their discussions of treatment with patients so that options and possible outcomes are clearly defined. Called the "shared decision model," this approach is based on a solid foundation.

> Academic research has suggested that when doctors share hard information about the risks and benefits of different treatment options, it can affect patients' decisions. Patients tend to choose less-aggressive treatments but still end up with similar outcomes and are more satisfied with their care. (Leonhardt, 2009, p. 37)

Changing the health care system to make this kind of mutual participation happen on a regular basis means consistently reviewing health care practices to eliminate the procedures that don't work. It is also necessary to be mindful of the kinds of support required in the home and the community to make these treatments successful. It is important to note that communities that are ethnically and economically diverse may not be able to create the outcomes that are found in a homogeneous community such as Salt Lake City, Utah (Leonhardt, 2009, p. 45). In addition, populations that are poor and underserved may also present with more multi-disease situations than in better-off communities. The upper-middle-class suburban community may have a healthier population than the low-income urban community and this fact, suggested in Chapter 1, must be taken into account in constructing chronic care service systems. In sum, what drives quality care for patients is the recognition of what could work in a given community.

Furthermore, the current payment system nationwide, based on fee-for-service, is one that encourages providers to do the extra and perhaps unnecessary procedure or test. A system such as Medicare that converts from a fee-for-service system and now pays a bundled fee for the treatment of a person with a chronic illnesses or surgery who enters a hospital stands a fighting chance of reducing costs and unnecessary procedures. The care would also involve incentives to keep people from being rehospitalized since the costs of that admission would be borne by the providers. Having some financial accountability or some "skin in the game" can make a difference in how medicine is practiced.

There is some history to the idea of accountability for medical practices when it comes to supplying chronic care. As presented in a story on National Public Radio on January 4, 2010, sent from the California station KQED, Sarah Varney identified the Redlands Family Practice as having a 26-year history of providing primary, specialty, and hospital care for patients with chronic illnesses for a fixed monthly payment. Called global payment, these funds were designed to cover all of the patient's medical and hospital costs based on the health condition of the patient. Surpluses were to remain with the providers and if there were cost overruns, the partners in the venture were to absorb the costs. To make sure that patients with multiple chronic illnesses were doing well, monthly visits to the primary care physician were required. Hospitalized patients were followed closely so they could make a smooth transition back to their homes and not become hospitalized again. Monthly reviews by primary care physicians of referrals to specialists were made and the economies found in the Redlands Family Practice added up to their spending 15 percent less than the regional average.

The chronic care model, as described in seven case studies by Robert A. Berenson of the Urban Institute, requires a new payment methodology that takes a detour around the cast iron fee-for-service system that is in place both in private and public insurance. Berenson (2006) states that

> chronic care management would be better supported with per patient per month (PPPM) payments, permitting the recipient organization to allocate staff and other resources, determine the appropriate mix of office and home visits, devise patient education and self-management protocols, and configure telephonic and Web-based communications. The PPPM payment amounts could be adjusted for underlying health status. (p. 8)

Berenson, in a later Web-posted article with Peter V. Lee and John Tooker, loses the PPRM approach, probably because it would require complete conversion to a health maintenance organization arrangement for all of Medicare. Lee, Berenson, and Tooker (2009) make an even stronger argument for the accountable care organization model, but clearly based on getting rid of the piece-rate approach to payment found in much of health care today.

> the current model of fee-for-service payments undercompensate evaluation and management services as compared with procedures and technical services, do a poor job of providing incentives to clinicians for collaboration, do not improve efficiency, are not focused on quality and outcomes, and do little to encourage wellness and prevention. Yet these fee-for-service payments could serve as the building blocks for setting payments for some of the alternative payment approaches, if the fee-for-service payments are used to determine the element of bundled payments or the component parts of payments for medical homes or accountable care organizations (ACOs).

Creating a workable team where doctors and hospitals seek improvement in quality so that patients, particularly the elderly, maintain or gain independence is a challenge. It also involves making it possible to point to cost reductions in the delivery of medical services. The Commonwealth Fund, seeking to create a high performance health system, has supported the study of the Massachusetts-based Mount Auburn Cambridge Independent Practice Association (IPA) and its partnership with Mount Auburn Hospital to negotiate with health plans to formulate an adequate capitation budget that is risk based, meaning that the IPA and the hospital are responsible for complete cost of patients' care. The budget is based on several factors, including

> Previous cost and utilization experience applied to the demographics (age and gender) and health conditions of the patient population (using a risk-adjusted methodology called diagnostic care groups), 2) projected cost trends, and 3) estimated cost savings to be achieved from care management activities. The IPA and hospital maintain reinsurance that assumes payment for catastrophic cases reaching a high-dollar (stop-loss) threshold. (Commonwealth Fund, 2010, p. 2)

This kind of initiative, found in demonstration and pilot programs and advocacy, was noticed by the writers of both the House and Senate health reform bills and there are incentives in the Affordable Care Act (PPACA) of 2010 that will encourage the creation of accountable care organizations (ACO), permitting health care providers to align payments for Medicare patients so that all of the participants will benefit financially. Connecting the key players should make it possible for costs for Medicare to come down over the next decade. The ACO is the financial platform for the patient-centered medical home, to be discussed shortly, for people with chronic illnesses. Astoundingly, Republican members of Congress, who are also doctors, find the funding of ACOs to be to their liking, even when they regard the rest of PPACA as bringing socialism to our fair land (Reichard, 2010a).

Some regional collaborative arrangements, where there is a history of sharing responsibilities, have been established to prepare for federal funding that will be available in 2011. Five hospitals, clinics, and other health care providers in New Hampshire have established an ACO to focus on prevention and health maintenance that will promote the avoidance of costly hospital admissions (Ramer, 2010). Collaboration in the Granite State promotes the management of the patient's condition going forward and uses information technology to identify patients who are at risk for hospitalization or visits to the emergency departments.

To make ACOs more understandable, many health care organizations have joined learning collaboratives, including start-ups sponsored by the American Medical Group Association (AMGA), so that health care organizations can learn from each other and be better at planning and implementing ACOs. Since some health care organizations have established the legal framework for their participation as an ACO, they are separated from those organizations that need to establish themselves as legally entitled to serve patients as an ACO (Klein, 2010, p. l).

Some of the existing programs, such as the St. John's Health System in Springfield, Missouri, have focused on ways of improving communication between providers and patients and between different kinds of providers, such as primary care and emergency department physicians (Klein, 2010, p. 2). Since the United States ranks fairly low internationally on several key measures related to patient centeredness, including the ease by which patients were "able to contact the doctor's office by phone and ask about a health problem during regular business hours" and have doctors explain medical issues in a way that they can understand, accountable care organizations should make a difference in improving communication between providers and their patients (Davis, Schoen, and Stremikis, 2010, p. 9)

ACOs that enhance communication could also improve the quality of care and the outcomes as well, not just save money for Medicare and private insurers. A good example of how this might work through enhanced coordinated care is what is happening at the Everett Clinic in the state of Washington. The multispecialty medical group with 300 physicians participated in the Medicare Physician Group Practice Demonstration. The Everett Clinic also entered into a special agreement with the aircraft manufacturer, the innovative Boeing Corporation, one of the major employers in the northwest, expanding on the idea of a nurse coordinator at the workplace.

> The clinic . . . implemented a care model that intensified primary care-services with patients with complex chronic conditions. The program provides these patients with psychosocial and behavioral health services. A nurse case manager plays a key role by planning visits, interviewing patients, and helping to facilitate weekly team rounding by the physician, care manager, and the pharmacist to discuss patient progress. The program saved Boeing 20 percent after program costs and case management fees, primary by reducing hospitalizations and emergency department visits. (Klein, 2010, p. 2)

Reducing spending is clearly one of the goals of creating an ACO and the payment reforms that induce these results are clearly important if we are going to rein in the cost of care in the United States. Measurement of whether and how the ACO system creates positive outcomes for patients and providers is also essential and needs to be done in a way that does not establish burdensome demands on the time of physicians and other health care professionals. Fisher and Shortell (2010) advocate the use of "longitudinal approaches to measurement that capture patient-reported health outcomes, the degree to which care was aligned with patients well-informed preferences and total cost of care" (p. 1715).

Some advocates of a better way to provide chronic care have taken a more episodic approach than the PPPM, which is really based on the Health Maintenance Organization way of financing care. ACOs, it is argued, cannot function unless there is a bundled payment approach. In an advocacy article on collective accountability and bundled Medicare payments, Hackbarth, Reischauer, and Mutti (2008) call for financing policies that will make for better value for the money that is spent on chronic care.

> Under a bundled payment approach Medicare would pay a single provider entity (comprising a hospital and its affiliated physicians) a fixed amount intended to cover the costs of providing a full range of Medicare-covered services delivered during the episode. (p. 3)

There is anecdotal process evidence from the Mount Auburn IPA case study, previously discussed in this chapter, that successful programs are built on medical home models within ACOs that address the needs of patients who are most likely to be hospitalized without a coordinated care plan. This requires the presence of an infrastructure that supports care management, as found in the following description.

> [P]atients are stratified based on their risk of poor outcomes as identified by their physician, a review of clinical data, or at hospital discharge. Patients at highest risk, such as those with severe chronic conditions such as congestive heart failure or uncontrolled diabetes, may receive home visits by a nurse practitioner (NP), under contract to the IPA, who provides intensive patient and family education, supports medication adherence, and helps prevent hospital admissions or readmissions. NPs also visit patient undergoing rehabilitation in skilled nursing units to help them make a timely and successful recovery, which can reduce a typical three-week length of stay to 12 to 14 days, depending on the patient's condition. (Using NPs rather than visiting nurses for this job allows for more timely care, since NPs can make medical decision "on

the spot" within the scope of their licenses.) Patients with less severe conditions or who make improvement receive periodic calls from nurse case managers employed by the IPA. (Commonwealth Fund, 2010, p. 2)

Does the infrastructure exist, even in large medical practices, to support an ACO? Research conducted by Diane R. Rittenhouse and her colleagues (2008) on medical groups suggests that there is still a way to go when it comes to finding what is called the medical home for patients with chronic illnesses. Using data from the 2006–2007 National Study of Physician Organizations, they sought out whether the principal components of coordinated and comprehensive care were available in these medical groups. They surveyed 1,162 organizations and found that only 32 percent of the 291 physician-directed medical practices that claimed to have the principal components of patient-centered medical homes actually had primary care teams. Additionally, electronic access to specialist referral notes, pharmacy electronic coordination, and nurse care managers were reported in less than half of the medical groups surveyed. Moreover, while more than half of the groups had a diabetes registry, a way to flag patients with serious chronic conditions, this was not the case for patients with asthma, congestive heart failure, and depression—all serious medical conditions that can require interventions to prevent hospitalization. Clearly, there was a mountain to climb in the way of building appropriate primary care to get where other countries, such as Denmark with its patient-centered primary care, are when it comes to how to deal with chronic care.

Primary care works best when it is thoroughly integrated with specialty care delivery and has the support of a care management system as well as electronic medical record system. A case study conducted by the Commonwealth Fund in 2010 on the Bronx-based Montefiore Medical Center demonstrated that despite serving a vulnerable population with 80 percent of revenues derived from Medicare and Medicaid, payers that are not as generous as commercial insurers, Montefiore was able to (1) extend access to primary care widely into the community and (2) perform care management in a targeted way. With the medical center and its physicians assuming financial risk, there were notable improvements in care delivery (Chase, 2010a).

The patient-centered medical home was adopted to increase access to primary care and to reduce visits to the emergency department (ED). The Montefiore Medical Center applied for Medical Home designation to the National Committee for Quality Assurance and if certified, New York State Medicaid will pay an enhanced rate for its primary care practices. This integrated care delivery system has already improved diabetes care through collaboration between upper level management, clinicians, and staff across the system, including nutritionists and health educators. Rates of glycemic control at outpatient settings went beyond standardized yardsticks. Asthma care also improved and fewer children were hospitalized or were treated in the ED.

Keeping discharged elderly patients out of hospitals and EDs was also part of the goals of Montefiore, accomplished in 2009 by having nurses make phone calls to patients. Through this effort at improving transition to the home, nurses were able to locate gaps in care and supply patient education, resulting in a reduction in the 30-day readmission rate from 19.9 percent to 13.2 percent (Chase, 2010b, p. 12).

Being able to do tests remotely also enhanced chronic care. The use of telemedicine in the home became a standard way to monitor Montefiore patients with chronic diseases. Locating problems early through this advanced technology was an advantage in care coordination and limited the need for rehospitalization.

Finally, while there is strong interest in the United States in pursuing the remaking of chronic care via the accountable care organization model, there is some caution demonstrated on the part of both health care providers and insurers. Providers, often hospitals, are concerned that they might be accused of price fixing to stifle competition when they enter into negotiations with insurance companies. The antitrust laws of the nation have to be considered when providers join up to deliver services only where private insurers are concerned and not when Medicare or Medicaid is in the picture. Indeed, antitrust laws are of concern when there is no public benefit from these partnerships so long as it does not paralyze markets. Alternatively, insurers are wary of providers banding together and leveraging their resources through ACOs to get better rates. These questions were posed at a meeting on October 5, 2010, where providers and insurers met with representatives from the Federal Trade Commission, the Centers for Medicare and Medicaid Services, and the Department of Health and Human Services to establish guidance for the formation of ACOs (Gold and Galewitz, 2010a). The meeting drew more than 300 representatives from all parts of the health care industry, including representatives from the National Community Pharmacist Association, monitoring device maker associations, and manufacturers of medical imaging and radiotherapy, along with hospital and physician group practices. The health care interests that are on the supply side were concerned that ACOs, with the emphasis on cost containment, would shrink their market share by encouraging less prescribing, testing, and screening. The representatives from these special interests expressed their interest as attempting to make sure that patients received all the care required (Gold and Galewitz, 2010b).

Change from the point of view of suppliers is always inappropriate, unless they start to consider that with many newly insured Americans by 2014 there will be many more patients for whom to fill prescriptions, monitor, and screen. Perhaps doctors and other health care providers will be kept so busy with the new patient base that the idea of doing any unnecessary activities will be a thing of the past. Hopefully, these newly emerging ACOs will be established to promote patient-centered medical home, sometimes called advanced primary care, the subject of the next chapter.

# 4

# The Patient-Centered Medical Home

The idea of having a doctor follow a patient through time, during periods of need and periods where little intervention is required, is at once both old-fashioned and modern. The image of the general practitioner with horse and buggy implies that house calls are made and the family history is known to the savvy provider who can tip the balance in the patient's favor. The modern side of the doctor who is there for the patient is found in the team of advanced practice providers such as the nurse practitioner who can make the care coordination for the frail elderly person seamless. The team approach means that the doctor who heads the team may be less directly responsible for patients and less responsive to them than a subordinate who can make a home visit and work with the family and friends who make up the circle of concern. Alternatively, the doctor can be summoned quickly to make a house call or when patients can be seen in the doctor's office if conditions require it. With this level of chronic care in place, hospital admissions and emergency department visits are the last resort. If chronic care is to work, it has to manage to nip in the bud serious declines in the health of the person, usually through the delivery of ambulatory care.

Paying primary care doctors to head a team that follows patients with chronic conditions, even when using state-of-the-art electronic medical record keeping, it would appear, often strikes the public narrative of the subject as a return to the old days when doctors had the time to get to know patients. When doctors charged modest fees, the technology was limited, and few patients had insurance, there were often strong ties that bound the caregiver and the care receiver. Today, with the vast development of specialty care, the primary care physician, who follows the medical home approach, also coordinates tests and specialty visits (Appleby, 2008). This is an old-fashioned approach with a contemporary twist, made somewhat easier by electronic medical records and the use of e-mail. This improvement in communication and planning is the foundation for a vast improvement over the fragmented care received by most patients with chronic illnesses, given that often they are not able to get their doctors to talk to each other or even reach their family practice physician. To what extent are these improvements in coordination appreciated by patients?

There are, strikingly, responses to the medical home by patients that suggest that those who are linked well to their primary care doctor do not want to have to be cared for by a team of providers. This kind of relationship may still exist, but with primary care physicians in short supply, I wonder how frequently that relationship is a reality. There also may be a substantial number of people in need of chronic care who cannot get linked up with either the team or the old-fashioned family doctor. Comments about what is missing when patients are in that fragmented situation are not easy to find. Comments about the patient-centered medical home are more readily available because the experience is new for many people and for reporters and columnists in the print and electronic media, this is the basis of a good story. Ironically, the story of inappropriate or badly designed care is not news.

In contrast, remade chronic care does spark comments from the recipients of it. There is a small set of unrepresentative comments to call on for some illumination on the issue. In written responses to a provocative article by Pauline W. Chen, MD, some bloggers, including Wayne Shipman, came to the defense of the patient-centered medical home. He weighed in with the following comments:

> Approximately 20 years ago, we enjoyed the benefits of a 'family practice' medical group in Derry, NH. Our two children were born under their care, as were both my and my wife's care. They had doctors, physician's assistants, nurses and a wonderful woman who could take blood samples for tests without you knowing it!
>
> It was without a doubt a model that works. We felt cared for, not by one doctor, but many, and always had access to trained care at appropriate levels.
>
> This is what the system needs to strive for. I don't want to see a doctor unless it's needed. If I can get a question answered by email, even better.
>
> If patients honored the doctor's time, and vice versa, we'd all be better for it. (Shipman, 2010)

While routine care is part of the mix, providers can act proactively, with the patient-centered team being able to prevent further deterioration rather than affect a cure. Hospital stays, even those of short duration, can often be followed by relapses. Note also—as mentioned earlier—for elderly patients who are leaving a hospital stay, the chances of returning within 30 days are one in five. The use of diagnostic related groups (DRGs) to determine the appropriate length of stay creates a financial incentive on the part of the hospital to not have the patient stay too long, since payments from commercial insurers and Medicare only cover a limited stay. The team approach then starts with patient-discharge planning, often required by hospital policy to be initiated within 24 hours following admission, and not only includes a determination that patients will have someone at home to look after them but they should have a plan in place for community-based monitoring of the patient's condition and to make sure that the patient receives medications or other interventions, such as simple test taking.

Yet, as suggested in Chapter 3, the payment system often does not put the doctor and the hospital on the same page. The current system of care encourages hospitals to discharge publicly and often privately insured patients from acute care facilities as early as possible or they face financial penalties. Indifference is often built into the reward structure—doctors don't get paid for follow-up of patients once they are discharged (Jauhar, 2009, p. D6). While it may appear only to be a cost concern and not something that should be dismissed lightly, this gap has prodded doctors into brainstorming about how, for example, to bundle the charges for a patient with thyroid cancer, including surgery, radiology, and endocrinology (Gawande, 2009). Lively debates ensue as each specialty attempts to get its fair share of the bundle. Without bundling of fees, many of the care coordination activities, not usually done by specialists, will not be supported. But there is, at least, a concept to pull all of this together and it is not new.

Designated the patient-centered medical home, the idea is that there is a location and a concerted effort to maintain the patient's lifestyle as much as possible, despite the possibility that there may be multiple diseases that the patient and providers must deal with at the same time. Consequently, the doctor and the team that delivers care for the chronically ill seek to reduce the likelihood that emergent problems will grow into an amalgam of raging acute disorders that require costly interventions and may be life threatening. Costly complications are the result of a failure to arrest decisively conditions that are sprouting so that hospitalizations can be avoided and the chronic care patient stays stable and therefore without the need of acute care. Providers need a new tool kit to accomplish a reversal of unsustainable costs and bad outcomes for patients and one is ready to build up to scale.

According to Bernstein, Chollet, Peikes, and Peterson (2010), a patient-centered medical home

> is a source of comprehensive primary care that provides services ranging from preventive care to management of chronic diseases. Medical homes promote a trusting ongoing relationship between patients and their primary care providers, helping patients to manage their health care better: Ideally, medical homes use integrated data systems and performance reporting to continuously improve access to and quality of care, as well as communication with patients and other providers. (p. 2)

The patient-centered medical home is designed to help prevent unnecessary use of emergency department facilities, but there may be deviant cases that don't fit neatly into this design. As noted in the following narrative, despite the gratitude expressed regarding the concern of the consulting cardiologist, there are limits to preventive interventions. Some exceptions apply, as in the case of this woman in her 60s that she accounted to me when she detailed her repeated experiences with emergency care.

> When I would have episodes of arythmia, my cardiologist, who is a model of patient centered care, would tell me to get myself over to the ER for cardioversion (electric shock) as quickly as possible, because I can't tolerate the standard medications, which cause my blood pressure to tank. Even the newest drug, Multaq, is ineffective when my heart gets going, and the only real treatment has been yet another heart ablation (I've had four).
>     The frequent trips to the ER (I've had 39 cardioversions), created a real confrontation between my Dr. and the head of the ER. Fortunately, the ablation seems to be working for now. I definitely have been a "frequent flyer," with a joking relationship with all the ER staff who man the early morning hours, but no amount of "case management" could correct the situation without more drastic treatment.

## ORIGINS OF THE MEDICAL HOME CONCEPT

This forward-thinking idea, which is anticipated to be a major part of delivery system reform as well as financing, is not all that new but comes initially from treating children with special health care needs. The concept of the medical home was introduced by the American

Academy of Pediatrics (AAP) in 1967. The first and simple step the AAP took in the fight against fragmentation of care was to seek a central location for a child's medical record. Later, AAP enriched the medical home concept to include features that would encourage continuous access and use of services by the family and where the services would be culturally effective, humane, and coordinated. Other professional medical associations such as the American Academy of Family Physicians, the American College of Physicians, and the American Osteopathic Association built on the original concept and have developed their own medical home concepts. Endorsed by these associations, the following principles describe the major features of the patient-centered medical home (Patient Centered Primary Care Collaborative, 2007).

- Personal physician
- Physician-directed medical practice
- Whole person orientation
- Quality and safety
- Enhanced access
- Payment recognizes value added by patient-centered medical home
- Care is coordinated and/or integrated

We will follow-up on the effectiveness and efficiency of the pediatric medical home model later in this chapter. First, there is need to recount how the pediatric patient-centered medical home evolved during the last 45 years. Registered nurses were trained to become advance practice nurses and then used in the 1970s to deliver accessible care to pediatric patients. When dealing with chronically ill children or adults who need to be hospitalized periodically for treatment or diagnostic work, nurse practitioners were especially good at explaining what kinds of tests or treatments patients would be undergoing, as well as how to manage at home. Confidence can be instilled in patients through the counseling and educational side of dispensing services. In so doing, nurse practitioners were able to reduce the disruptive effects of being rehospitalized or discharged from the hospitals. This kind of preventive mental health work was initiated in consultation with a supervising physician, sometimes with psychiatrists or psychiatric social workers.

In the following exchange, which took place in the early 1970s when I was doing field observation at a major medical center on the activities conducted by nurse practitioners and the development of their professional identities, a pediatric nurse practitioner (PNP) was able to explain to a child who was receiving home care that he was going back to the hospital on a temporary basis. This boy had been subject to a lengthy hospitalization for extensive reconstruction of his stomach and a return to the hospital could be traumatizing. He was going to be hospitalized for a short-term visit, for an endoscopic examination of the esophagus, and without the kind of preparation indicated in the exchange that follows below, the child might have believed that he was going into the hospital for a long stay.

**PNP:** I have something to tell you, Fred. You can come to the hospital to play, not to stay. The doctors are going to take an X-ray. Do you know what X-rays are?

**Fred:** X-rays?

**PNP:** It's a picture. You have to drink something to make the picture work. (Birenbaum, 1990, p. 92)

The use of the medical home model for the care of children who once died from such feared diseases such as leukemia but now survive calls for an emphasis on the whole person orientation in great detail. Suffice it to say that with children, personal development goes beyond the whole person orientation. Sometimes the developmental requirements go unrecognized when the child is in a life-risking situation, driven by the disease or diseases that are being treated. The multiple chronic conditions that the child often has to bear relate to the powerful treatments undergone. Once again, reporter Amy Docker Marcus, in a complex newspaper article on the life of an eight-year-old boy who received chemotherapy and radiation to stop his blood-based cancer in its tracks, notes also that this invasive treatment created enormous side-effects that affect the quality of life of the child. As we know, powerful interventions carry costs to the body.

This Natick, Massachusetts, child suffered dental problems, a side effect of the radiation, and needed cataract surgery to correct a condition resulting from the drugs that he took (Marcus, 2004b).

And there is more that caregivers must attend to. The new therapies reverse the odds of survival beyond five years for children and adults but increase their physical, emotional, and developmental needs. In some ways, these conundrums are indicators that the child is engaging in ordinary childhood experiences as well as the unusual. The whole person, as a member of the community, goes from being a collective project to one where there is ambiguity about how to treat them. There are many questions to consider when undergoing these life-extending therapies. Should Jack, now that he is out of danger and back in school, be treated like any other child and be subject to school discipline when he gets into a fight with another boy in his class? Should he be given growth hormones to help him be closer in stature to the other children of the same age in his neighborhood since radiation to the brain can stunt growth? Will he develop cognitive problems as a result of his chemotherapy (Marcus, 2004b)?

The emotional issues raised by Jack's survival are also in need of coordinated care in a patient-centered medical home. Children and adults change when engaged in these battles with cancer or when left with permanent disabilities. The evidence is strong, according to the President's Cancer Panel report (June 2004), that one in five children who survive cancer undergo posttraumatic stress disorder. While coping styles vary, parents are advised to create a scrapbook of the child's treatment experience, which can be used if, later in life, the person wants more detail on what happened to him or her as a youthful patient (Marcus, 2004b). Clearly, the scrapbook helps create continuity in a person's story in his or her battle to live with a chronic illness.

## PUTTING PATIENTS FIRST

Contemporary health care can be technologically impressive but often providers fail to consider the patient as partners in the care process. Coordinated care means that the patient as a person is respected and he or she is not just a collection of organs and systems that need servicing. The image of a passive patient simply visiting various specialists is transformed to one of a patient who is actively engaged in the planning and delivery of coordinated care. Consequently, the patient-centered medical home is also built around the idea of eliminating a fragmented care system that does not benefit the patient and is costly to maintain. Fragmentation promotes the duplication of services or the delivery of unnecessary services. A review of the services delivered in an uncoordinated fashion often reveals that tests are ordered and procedures performed for which there do not appear to be valid reasons. Sometimes there is the readying of expensive supplies that won't be needed for an operation, supplies that may be billed to the patient's account. When data are collected prior to and after the implementation of coordinated care, there are often clear savings found in expenditures for the care of people with multiple conditions.

Care coordination for children is also problematic when there are multiple disabling conditions, as reported in the analysis of cross-sectional data collected from interviews with parents of 3- to

17-year-olds in the 2005–2006 National Survey of Children with Special Health Care Needs (CSHCN). Bitsko and her colleagues (2009, p. S343) reported that parents of CSHCN with neurologic conditions were more likely than parents of children with other CSHCN to list unmet health needs for their child. But even more interesting was the finding that "the 2 subgroups with multiple conditions had the greatest unmet needs and dissatisfaction with care coordination" (p. S349). Clearly when care coordinators have to deal with multiple conditions, this opens the door to having to work with several specialists at the same time, providers who are impatient to get on to the next task and often not familiar with the idea of the medical home.

Results from the National Survey of Children with Special Health Care Needs, 2005–2006, suggest that there is far to go in the United States organizationally and financially to get the care children require from a patient-centered medical home. A little more than half of the families reporting (57.4%) said that they partner in decision making at all levels and are satisfied with the services they receive. Less than half of the parents interviewed (47.4%) said that the child with special health care needs received coordinated ongoing comprehensive care within a medical home. And, finally, only 41.2 percent of the parents of older children interviewed said that youth with special health care needs received the services they required to make transitions to all aspects of adult life, including adult health care, work, and independence (U.S. Department of Health and Human Services, *The National Survey of Children with Special Health Care Needs Chartbook 2005–2006*, 2008).

The chronic care model, discussed in Chapter 6 in detail with regard to adult patients, may face even more challenges when dealing with comorbidities found in children. Just as families are challenged by the child's multiple medical and disabling conditions, the care coordination services are equally subject to challenges. The patient-centered medical home, when it counts, can be found wanting for children and their families and may even require a great deal of effort on the part of independent adults.

## PARTICIPATING IN THE PATIENT-CENTERED MEDICAL HOME

The patient-centered medical home is designed to meet the needs and choices of patients who want to contribute to their own care plan and who aspire also to avoid or reduce their inpatient hospital care. It is an alternative to tertiary care, the complex and technologically sophisticated interventions that are done in university-affiliated acute care hospitals. Participation means avoiding passivity while receiving medical care and allows for patient autonomy, knowing that more care is sometimes less effective than coordinated care.

Sometimes coordinated care is one-dimensional because of the emphasis on focusing on a single disease. The woman quoted earlier, a person who responded to the issues raised by a narrow focus and who I corresponded with in preparation for this book, mentioned that care coordination was supposed to be performed by her primary care physician as part of the managed care plan that her employer furnished for staff. But the care was less than required.

> After my first bouts with atrial fibrillation and my first ablations, I was referred to a program, which took about six months to complete, where I received monthly calls from a nurse, based out in Tennessee. I was not sure what category they put me in, as the program was supposed to be either for coronary artery disease or congestive health failure, neither of which I have.
>
> I quickly found out that the nurse assigned to me knew much less about my condition—mitral stenosis and atrial fibrillation and atrial flutter—than I did. Other than an initial interview about my other lists of diagnoses, she never asked anything about them. Each month I would report to her that I was still struggling to keep my weight under control, and then we would talk about my grandchildren.

Clearly this experience was disappointing and this person with multiple chronic diseases turned to the Internet for better guidance than was available through her managed care plan. Sometimes the care coordination is user friendly with face-to-face help available. There are also some good reasons, given the nature of the chronic care required, for a specialist to be the care coordinator, rather than the primary care physician or even a physician extender.

Coordinated care often works so well that the patient may not know what profession the provider represents, as mentioned by a *New York Times* blogger, who saw a physician assistant without knowing it. In this story, Ruth (2010) "found her very knowledgeable and interested in me, and I enjoyed the visit. My doctor didn't miss a beat when I saw her about a month later. She had read the notes and knew what had been done, so it was seamless."

The concept of a home implies a warm and cozy place, perhaps with the aroma of baked apples offering a welcoming touch, as well as a technologically driven approach to care. When the concern is for the patient's safety and dignity, it is possible for the medical team to be less invasive in the patient's life with the care that is delivered. There are patients for whom the medical-home model won't work. The person who is declining mentally, as in the case of dementia, may not be a good candidate for self-management of the intense requirements of diabetes.

Disease management, when the goal is optimizing the patient's well-being rather than addressing cost issues, as in the case of type 2 diabetes, means that effective communication becomes central to the delivery of quality care in the patient-centered medical home (PCMH). Four professional associations representing various subspecialists, according to the Commonwealth Fund, define core features of PCMH as the following:

- Improving access and communication through policies such as open scheduling and e-mail communication between doctors and patients
- Using integrated data systems to streamline care
- Facilitating patient and family engagement and culturally sensitive care
- Adopting advanced clinical information systems to reduce errors and expand the physician's access to critical information and guidelines

Sometimes people with comorbidities are able to see the virtues of this approach because necessity makes these goals count. MM, yet another blogger, seems to touch most of the bases in the following extensive comments.

> I like the computer in the doctor's office. Yes, it's a delicate balance between looking at the patient and typing up notes.
>     But I have a complex medical history and take several medications. When I see any doctor within my system, they can log in and look at my patient records, with all the comments (typed—not written in a scrawl) right there. The nurses always check to make sure the medication list is up to date, and since they do change regularly, that is important.
>     I recently had a doctor's visit that lasted 1.5 hours and which involved quite a bit of history taking and explanation. Had the doctor had to write it all out by hand, half of it would not have made it to the page at any given time and it would have been harder to go back and edit to give a more accurate picture as new information was obtained from me. In a later visit with a neurologist, he pulled up the history, read it, and we quickly moved on to figuring out the problem without rehashing everything that was said in the previous visit. (2010)

Some health care delivery systems have attempted to put these principles into action and see if the outcomes demonstrate the value of this approach. The Seattle, Washington, based Group Health Co-operative conducted a two-year pilot project with patients in a medical-home prototype that examined the quality of care, clinician burnout, and total costs, as compared to patients and their caregivers seen by this program who were not in the medical home pilot. Chronic care management included the use of electronic registries, health maintenance reminders, and best practices alerts to staff. The care team engaged in motivational interviewing and used negotiation skills to keep patients compliant with treatment regimens. In collaboration with patients, care plans were developed to guide patients and the care team. A strong emphasis was placed on patient self-management, including group visits, behavior change programs, and workshops for people with chronic illnesses (Reid et al., 2010, p. 837).

The actively engaged patient is considered by current designers of patient-centered medical homes to be a central partner in the chronic care process. Getting patients engaged is often dependent on finding out what level of engagement patients are at when they enter these programs. At the University of Oregon, "To measure individuals' skill and competence in managing their health, as well as to gauge their beliefs about their role in managing their health, [Judith] Hibbard and her colleagues developed the Patient Activation Measure (PAM)—a statistical measure used when precision and consistency are critical—based on a 13 question survey that assesses the patient's confidence in chronic disease self-management" (Chase, 2010b, pp. 1–2). Once available, the PAM results can be used to determine what level of coaching a patient requires or whether a clinical intervention is necessary. The PAM is utilized to take action to prevent a readmission, to identify patients who are noncompliant, and to identify gaps in care related to a patient's lack of knowledge, ability, or motivation (Chase, 2010b, p. 3).

Although few who supplied feedback on their care experiences were familiar with the term "medical home," patient satisfaction was evident when positive comments were made about the ease of communication via e-mail, reminders about making appointments, and virtual visits with members of the care coordination team (Meyer, 2010, p. 846). There were also money-saving features as well. During the study period, using clinical and administrative data, the research team found that the prototype clinic outperformed the other providers according to several indicators. And while primary care costs were more expensive within the pilot program, the patients at the prototype clinic made fewer emergency department visits and had fewer inpatient admissions (Reid et al., 2010, p. 838).

For some clinicians attempting to redeploy via the patient-centered medical home so there can be a better way to deliver primary care, there have been surprising learning experiences when it comes to patient perceptions. One unanticipated finding from a national demonstration project in transforming primary care practices into patient-centered medical homes was the confusion experienced by patients and their families. First, the concept of a medical home was clearly mistaken by laypeople for other practices such as home care or group homes. But most importantly patients were not comfortable with change and how to navigate the new system, with its multiple providers and the paperless office.

> Some felt displaced as they see the old one-to-one doctor-patient interactions replaced with one-to-three or one-to-four relationships involving not only the doctor but also a whole host of other providers. As offices switched from paper-based to electronic medical records, other patients reacted to the distracted clinicians who seemed more focused on learning the new computer system than on listening to them. Satisfaction fell because, like my friend, few patients were cognizant of, much less involved in, the changes going on around them. (Chen, 2010)

Second, patients come with histories that can help predict reactions to the medical home model. It would be useful to determine whether patients with chronic illnesses were more or less unhappy with the new system than healthy patients being told they are now being cared for in a patient-centered medical home. Additionally, are patients with multiple hospitalizations or emergency room visits more or less comfortable with the new delivery system than patients who had chronic illnesses but were not at risk for acute outbreaks? I anticipate that the data collection effort and subsequent reports on outcomes related to this national demonstration project will help to answer these questions. Any attempt to create team-based, comprehensive, and preventive care cries out for this kind of analysis.

Another one of Dr. Chen's bloggers LizCA (Chen, 2010) pointed to the conditions under which a patient-centered medical home would be effective and a waste of time.

> This could work, if there is ONE PERSON at the center who is coordinating everything.
> 
> It really doesn't matter to me if it's a doctor or a nurse practitioner, but I want one person who has the time to meet me, to read my darn test results and to coordinate with other practitioners.
> 
> But if the result is medical care by vague bureaucratic groups, a lot of info will get lost along the way. As it is, my quite wonderful primary

care provider barely has time to really look at my test results or do any extended follow-up, as she is only paid for office visits, and a quite paltry sum for that.

There are costs for providers who make the transition to the patient-centered medical home model. Experience with conversion from solo or group primary care practice to patient-centered medical homes comes with an emotional price for physicians. Practice patterns and professional self-images change. Communication with the surrounding professional neighborhood can also be daunting.

> Physicians in specialty practice have little incentive to communicate with medical-homes to help them coordinate care and might also resist efforts to manage referrals to specialty services.... Consumers may resist what they perceive as restricting their access to specialists or particular services and facilities. (Bernstein, Chollet, Peikes, and Peterson, 2010, p. 2)

Some primary care physicians have found the alternative reaction from patients, particularly where chronic care management can be conducted largely in the patient's home. Steven H. Landers (2010, pp. 1–4) states that it is over-determined that home visits for patients with multiple chronic illnesses are the wave of the future. He identifies five factors driving this trend:

1. An aging population and the increasing prevalence of chronic illnesses
2. The risks of falls, dizziness, and rashes for older patients during hospital stays
3. Advances in miniaturization and portability of equipment combined with remote monitoring and long-distance care
4. The ethos of consumerism, which calls for more convenience for patients
5. The financing of in-home rehabilitation and infusion services often makes home care the least expensive alternative and limits opportunities for other providers in hospitals to pile on unnecessary services.

Landers offers the reader a feel for how health care is the home goods.

> I work in my patients' homes, using a cellular broadband connection to the same electronic record system used by my colleagues in offices and hospitals. I learn practical information about my patients' medications, management of chronic illnesses, and nutrition and check in on how their caregivers are coping. Patients often see the home visit as a gesture of caring, and many of my older patients express nostalgia for an era when house calls were common. (p. 1)

The precedent for home visits came from the innovations established during the 1970s at pediatric departments that were trying to get children with serious chronic illnesses and who had become almost permanent residents in wards back to their families. The idea was that these "boarders," as they were designated by pediatricians and nurse practitioners, were more likely to thrive better with their families than in a hospital bed. By teaching parents how to do various procedures that nurses would do in hospitals, these innovative programs increased the odds that the child would thrive and also keep up with their educational requirements via home schooling (Birenbaum, 1990, p. 92). What was offered 40 years ago was primitive because the truly portable technology that Dr. Landers raves about was not yet invented. (I can attest to the difficulties of making a home visit with what was called a "portable" EKG machine, a device that was quite heavy to carry, when as a medical sociologist in the field I accompanied a pediatric nurse practitioner on a home visit in a Bronx tenement and walked up four flights of stairs.) There is a need to rethink the medical home today, particularly for special and vulnerable populations with lifelong conditions.

As noted earlier, specialists can become accountable for care in the patient-centered medical home. There are occasions when the primary care physician, well versed in medical home thinking, will designate a specialist to be responsible for management of maintaining the medical home. Like a good neighbor, the specialist will take over from the primary care provider in the medical home under special circumstances. These transitions are done to provide evident-based management in a fully accountable way, with full control over management tasks and timely communication of recommendations and changes in therapies undertaken. Even with the specialist as primary care coordinator, the PCMH practice is responsible for the patient's whole person care. This may be a necessary strategy to maintain quality care over time when diseases flare up intermittently, such as when Crohn's disease becomes active (Greenlee, 2010).

## BUILDING SYSTEMS OF CARE FOR CHILDREN WITH SPECIAL HEALTH CARE NEEDS

With approximately one in every seven children under the age of 18 in the United States having special needs based on increased risk of having conditions that require health and related services beyond those required by children generally, it is no wonder that they have been a target of concern of the Maternal and Child Health Bureau, a Public

Health Service branch of the Department of Health and Human Services, nested in the Health Resources and Services Administration.
There may also be increased risks for secondary conditions. All in all,
and it should come as no surprise to the reader, children with special
health care needs (CSHCN), while a mere 14 percent of the child population, account for 42 percent of the expenditures on medical care for
children.

And it also follows that experts on CSHCN advocate that these children "receive coordinated ongoing comprehensive care within a
medical home" (Kogan, Strickland, and Newacheck, 2009, p. S334).
Today, there is an inverse relationship between need and access to
the medical home. Adequate care coordination was least likely to be
found among children with the most severe conditions and they were
less likely than those with less severe restrictions to have a medical
home or receive other required services (e.g., transition, preventive
care). In addition, the opportunity costs for parents were greater if
there was poor care coordination. Those parents with an adequate
care-coordination plan in place were less likely to report giving up
employment or reducing their hours as well as having higher out-of-
pocket costs. Good care coordination may also prevent the child from
being exposed to further risks and limit future consequences as far as
chronic illness is concerned. This proactive approach or preventive
intervention has been advocated by pediatricians for decades and
there is a sense that we are approaching a new dawn for children with
serious chronic illnesses.

Improving child outcomes may be within our reach through the
expansion of well-designed programs that could be supported
through health care reform. Laraque and Sia (2010) have argued for
the need to better understand the components of what they call the
family centered medical home, one that has all the nonmedical elements that a child needs as well as access to evidence-based treatment,
as needed.

> The obvious threat to providing primary care would be the inability to
> ensure coordination of services within a longitudinal relationship by a
> group of child health professionals with specific knowledge about the
> management of her complex problems. (p. 2408)

Despite the promise of this approach, advocates for medical homes
for CSHCN are somewhat humbled by the fact that what is perceived
as the foundation of community care has been rarely subject to systematic evaluation. The evidence to show that this intervention is a

decisive benefit to the child, the parents, and the payers for medical care, which was sought systematically, does not match the clear benefits found in the literature on medical homes for adults.

There was moderate support for the medical home model after 33 journal articles were reviewed to determine whether there was evidence to support the medical home model in its entirety. There were positive outcomes found in terms of "family centeredness, effectiveness, timeliness, health status, and family functioning" (Homer et al., 2008, p. e2934). The medical home construct goes far beyond these outcomes to include a reduction in costs to the health care system, developmental outcomes, and the functional status of the child; these results could be demonstrated through random controlled trials, where the traditional forms of care are compared against programs with sophisticated care coordination, under the direction of qualified primary care providers.

Some of these innovations work closely with existing delivery systems founded on a subtle mix of high technology and care coordination. Programs such as the Maternal and Child Health Bureau's Healthy Tomorrows, which funds 10 programs around the country through grants, has established in Philadelphia, Pennsylvania, "Baby-steps to Health," a transition support for medically and socially at-risk infants and families going from the Neonatal Intensive Care Unit (NICU) to the Pediatric Center at the Albert Einstein Medical Center. Lubricating this transition is a patient liaison, the staff member who becomes the primary support for the baby's caregiver even before they leave the NICU and remaining in the picture until the family no longer needs this intervention. And the patient liaison is always available to answer the parents' questions (Pulse, 2010, p. 11).

Yet I am reminded by a parent of a grown child with a disability, one with lots of experience with the U.S. health care system, that not all patient liaisons have the ability to be of assistance to stressed parents. Parents may resent the presence of another person to deal with, often perceived as barriers to contact with the real sources of help. The help that is appreciated is often extremely focused, with immediate results and directly reduced stress. Sometimes expressive exchanges get in the way of the instrumental needs, including learning the signs of distress as perceived by parents.

Learning how to avoid complications is considered important by parents. There are some hopeful signs that older children with asthma can benefit from intensive instruction to parents and child by physicians to make sure that prescriptions drugs that had to be taken daily were there as well as the more child-friendly inhaler. Following the completion of a 12-point asthma questionnaire, one Bronx parent found that her daughter was breathing more easily and making few visits to the Emergency Department because there were fewer flare-ups. Ms. Fria, a mother of four, acknowledged that it was easy to forget the child's medication, "But if you have a regular doctor who sits with you and makes sure you understand what's going on, it really helps. My message is knowledge is power" (Rabin, 2010b).

These positive outcomes are not free but result from carefully designed public expenditures. Medical homes, preventive dental care, and greater satisfaction with care, according to this national survey, were more likely to be found in progressive states that supported these services and helped to reduce the burdens on families. In addition, many of the elements of medical homes are found in federally supported and qualified health clinics in low income neighborhoods (Friedberg, Coltin, Safran, Dresser, and Schnieder, 2010, p. 938).

## MATCHING THE PAYMENT SYSTEM TO THE SERVICES DELIVERED

The previously discussed Group Health demonstration project in Seattle was grounded in a health professional team orientation that adhered to evidence-based practices and established long-term relationships between patients and providers. In addition, the health care team supplied comprehensive and coordinated care. To scale this up so that large numbers can be served, the payment systems have to reward these activities (Reid et al., 2010, p. 842).

How is the patient-centered medical home paid for? Recruiting providers is important and there need to be incentives for physicians to do PCMH. However, few new graduates from medical colleges go into primary care. Medical school debt and the long hours for limited financial rewards discourage future doctors from becoming the care coordinators that are critically required for there to be a shift from acute care to the PCMH. The need is urgent because, as noted earlier, Medicare, the popular federal insurance program for seniors and some people with disabilities, does not create sufficient financial incentives for care coordination. Some of the Medicare Advantage Plans, the enriched managed care plans for Medicare beneficiaries that requires voluntary enrollment, do promote disease management. By virtue of the capitation payment system that supports them, Medicare

Advantage plans provide care coordination and seek to keep patients from being rehospitalized. However, Medicare beneficiaries face a dilemma when they consider going with one of the Advantage plans. Since signing up for Medicare Advantage may mean losing one's long-term provider who may not be part of the Medicaid Advantage plan, these managed care plans have attracted the well rather than the sick. It goes without saying that the administrators of these plans are happy to serve the well and avoid the sick, popularly known as cherry picking.

Many innovations in care coordination come from the flexibility of states when it comes to employing their Medicaid programs to improve service delivery. Since Medicaid, the means-tested federal-state program, has a long experience with care management and co-ordination for severely chronically ill and disabled populations, there are more state-generated and federally approved payment methodol-ogies available for care coordination than in Medicare. Senior citizens who are poor may be eligible for both Medicare and Medicaid. Some of the components of the Patient Protection and Affordable Care Act, when they come online in 2013 and 2014, furnish many incentives both for pilot studies in medical homes and also to improve the Medi-care payment structure so that more physicians will be willing to work in primary care.

Clearly, the direction for all payment for care when it comes to chronic diseases is to move toward a bundled payment system that will redirect medical efforts toward keeping the patient well or at least stabilized and lowering the dependency on acute care interventions. The flaws in the current split payment system are evident. Many patients do not get to see their doctor during the first 30 days follow-ing hospital discharge, whether because of a lack of access or a percep-tion that the doctor's services are not required so soon after discharge. Most importantly, under current Medicare statutes, doctors cannot be paid to help reduce hospital stays. Bonuses for hospitals to lower readmission rates will need to be shared with attending physicians who will seek or be attracted to financial incentives to do appropriate follow-up for their formerly hospitalized patients (Jauhar, 2009, p. D6). As noted earlier, Medicaid rates make serving those patients in large numbers unattractive to physicians in the community.

Dr. Sandeep Jauhar, a cardiologist on suburban Long Island in New York State, argues that gainsharing is required if we are to reduce the cost of health care where it counts—by offsetting hospital readmis-sions by establishing the medical home to monitor and care for the patient with a serious chronic illness. As he states, "Our system needs to provide inducements to decrease the amount of health care, especially with the current incentives that encourage overutilization" (2009, p. D6). Dr. Jauhar is in agreement with the Massachusetts Special Commission on the Health Payment System, which found little incentive to achieving positive results or for care coordination because of low financial margins for those services. The commission recommended the adoption of medical homes, with an emphasis on patient-centered care, primary care, and patient choice.

One way to reduce the amount of unnecessary health care delivered is to redirect resources from specialty care to primary care. The chronic care team would be part of the primary care provider's purview and doctors, ideally, would learn in medical school and in their training how to work in a team that is made up of professionals who support each other and respect what it is that each contributes to the patient's well-being. Medical schools have far to go with regard to achieving this objective. However, there is recognition within the profession of medicine of the importance of getting this kind of teaming going. A dialogue between primary-care physicians, sponsored by the *New England Journal of Medicine* in November 2008, deals with the issues that must be addressed to change the delivery system, including financing of chronic care (Perspectives, 2008, pp. 2636–2638). Still, the gap is closing through nationwide information-gathering efforts.

Scaling up is being promoted through federal data collection efforts. The Center for Medicare and Medicaid Services, the government unit that oversees these public health insurance programs, has developed a pilot project that by July 2010 will include 80,000 physicians to look at the variation in resources used to treat similar chronic conditions. Entitled resource use reporting, or RUR, this data collection system will determine the cost per episode of care for Medicare patients based on a fee-for-service payment system. Data collection will include the total costs of hospital service, skilled nursing care, home care, emergency department resource utilization, imaging, and durable medical equipment. This information collection project is clearly a broad-based effort to stimulate change in physician behavior, a necessary part of reining in health care costs, since it is estimated that doctors are accountable for 65 percent of the health care charges in the United States.

The RUR system is designed to wring savings from a system that encourages inefficient providers and to put the spotlight on and reward those physicians and hospitals that do things well and at reasonable cost. It is anticipated that the performance of some inexpensive interventions will reduce the need to hospitalize patients and the volume of unnecessary services. It is likely that evidence derived from this pilot project will lead to the creation of bundling and capitation as a form of payment. Ultimately, what may be needed to support this massive shift in how medicine is practiced is the creation of a remuneration system for doctors that is based on salaries exclusively, rather than fee-for-service payments, which encourages the generation of big-ticket interventions.

There is also a recognition in the health services research and policy community that hospitalized patients who come from previous residency in nursing facilities are largely Medicaid eligible and from the perspective of the management of the nursing home and state Medicaid programs, there is little incentive to lower spending through Medicare for hospital and skilled nursing home stays. Pilot projects such as the Home Value-Based Purchasing demonstration, designed to reduce Medicare payments for hospital stays by rewarding nursing homes, has some promise as well as creating opportunities to game the system via cherry picking of patients for avoiding hospital admission according to their profitability (Mor, Intrator, Feng, and Grabowski, 2010, p. 63).

## A PLETHORA OF PILOT PROGRAMS

There are many pilot programs that have been established in the United States, mostly on a much smaller scale than the RUR, to promote better care for chronic illness while reducing the use of hospitals and emergency departments. Multiple disease management is critical in these efforts along with recognition that many of the problems that lead to hospital admissions and emergency room visits are related to housing and other environmental factors. The thinking that goes into the design of some of these pilot programs in sociodemographically vulnerable neighborhoods suggest that the designers were familiar with some of the prospective studies presented in Chapter 1 on how low-income people respond through high-risk behavior to stresses better-off individuals are able to avoid.

Coordinated care is always the foundation of the pilot programs for those in vulnerable neighborhoods. A team created by the Camden Coalition of Healthcare Providers in New Jersey worked with patients with diabetes to make sure that patients checked their blood sugar and took their medications when indicated. The Camden team worked with an extremely low-income population that included people who were homeless and lived in shelters. As usual, the data from the local hospitals showed that one percent, or slightly more than 1,000 patients, accounted for 40,000 hospital or emergency department visits a year at the cost of $46 million (Campbell, 2009, p. 3). Thus, the "frequent flyers" of the community were the targets of this intervention.

The Garden-State team created a "medical home without walls" that dramatically reduced emergency service and hospital admission utilization from 61 to 37 per month and cut the charges in half to $531,000. This citywide program employed a nurse practitioner, a social worker, and a community health worker and was similar in results found in other pilot projects in other cities in terms of cost savings.

There are other strategies to change medical practices with difficult populations, as seen in the following description of a New York City pilot program. Starting with the idea that data are critical to locate people who need attention, the researchers and clinicians raised a fundamental but creative question: Is it possible to identify prospectively who among the members of the community are likely to become expensive users of health services later in life and then attempt to prevent that high utilization rate to occur? Researchers, lead by John Billings at the venerable Bellevue Hospital New York City, after building an algorithm—or a step-by-step procedure using computers to solve a problem—identified and predicted three to four years in advance that some community residents would emerge as heavy users of health services. The variables employed were a combination of social and behavioral characteristics (Raven, 2009).

During hospital admissions, extensive interviews were conducted with 50 algorithmically identified patients and their providers. The interviewers found high rates of substance use, mental illness, homelessness, social isolation, and chronic disease as well as poor options for post-discharge family care. To reverse the odds of their returning to the hospital and being readmitted, the directors of the pilot intervention enrolled 19 Bellevue Hospital patients and did intensive case management that was patient centered and designed to bridge the gap between the health system and the community. The intervention was customized for complex patients with unique yet predictable needs.

It may come as no surprise to readers that housing was a major service issue and was tackled as a first priority by a team of social workers and community-based managers. A similar observation was made by the directors of the Vermont Family 360 Support Project, a program designed to keep children with parents with disabilities by supplying "Peer Navigators" who provide support and system navigation (Holsopple, 2010). Enrollees in the Bellevue project were given various kinds of assistance to facilitate their living in the community, including but not exclusively such assistance as staff accompaniment of patients to medical and other appointments, cell-phone provision and support, and entitlement enrollment, e.g., Medicaid and Supplemental Security Disability Income. In a comparison of the 12 months prior to and the 12 months post-enrollment, the individuals in the program had 26 percent fewer emergency department visits and inpatient admissions decreased by 45 percent. Outpatient visits increased and total annual savings to Medicaid, because of the reduction in the use of expensive hospital based services, was an impressive $11,922 per patient per year (Raven, 2009).

Cost offsets in pilot studies, the policy analyst term for savings by providing less expensive alternative services, get attention beyond the confines of local areas where they were conducted. This pilot project evolved into a New York State Department of Health Chronic Illness Demonstration Project, focusing on helping patients at one of three New York City Hospitals by fielding staff who would furnish assistance in helping them find housing, transportation, and food and nutrition support, among several ways of meeting unmet needs. The expectation for this ongoing project, "Hospital to Home: We'll Meet You Where You Are," is to improve health and reduce admissions and costs for a three-year period in comparison with a control group. It is anticipated that this expanded pilot program will enroll 500–550 patients across three New York City municipal hospitals and medical centers.

Not all pilot projects that seek to divert formerly hospitalized patients from readmission are effective, but it is instructive to do a postmortem. Hudson Headwaters Health Network, in a rural location in the Adirondack Park area of New York State, used a transition care staff consisting of one hospital-based physician assistant and two ambulatory-based registered nurses to work with 301 patients for more than nine months. While patients in the experimental group, in a pre- and post-program comparison, gained a substantial amount of information about their conditions and how to identify warning signs and symptoms and the purposes of their medications, there were some notable setbacks. Patients had difficulties getting appointments with primary care physicians following discharge due to a shortage of primary care doctors in that rural area. In addition, the early results of the pilot showed no differences with regard to readmission rates for the intervention and the control group with both showing slightly more than 17 percent (Shannon, 2009).

Another approach to reducing hospital admissions and the lengths of stays is derived from the awareness of dangers for patients in hospitals that result from mismanaged care. There are accidental injuries and deaths that are preventable both through better practices in hospitals and the creation of a capacity to deliver quality care to patients in the community so they will not be readmitted to a hospital. The Maine Health Management Coalition is a coalition of 21 employers, 21 hospitals, 14 provider groups, and 5 health plans that seeks value-based payment for health care (Mitchell, 2009).

The work done via financial incentives redirected providers to seek lifestyle changes for the subjects in this pilot study. Not only does this "down-east" coalition create rewards for employees to seek out guidance on exercise and diet by eliminating copayments for visits to providers, but it also incentivizes providers by allotments that give them higher payments for nutrition/lifestyle support. It should be noted that these kinds of health maintenance visits are not necessarily with physicians and these nonphysician fees are quite modest. The Maine coalition is also developing a model that involves pilots for shared decision making, reducing readmissions, and the formation of patient-centered medical homes.

Aligning payments is the key to the success of these programs. Piloted in four states, the Prometheus payment model developed new payment methodologies for chronic care and will be expanded in 2010. (Those who remember classical Greek mythology note that Prometheus brought fire to human life, thereby promoting the advancement of civilization, a quest not too different from taming today's disjointed health care system.) The emphasis conceptually is on developing a bundled payment or a global fee system that accounts for all care related to a medical event. Providers gain by improving quality and lowering costs by avoiding possible complications. The health care industry is redirected to seeking value in services rather than volume, as in the case of a fee-for-service payment system (deBrantes, Rosenthal, and Painter, 2009). Patients are evaluated to determine the level of severity in each case so that providers will be compensated fairly and will thereby eliminate the avoidance of adverse risks or, once more in the language of private insurers, cherry picking.

Many of these efforts involve rethinking or remodeling health care and introducing a medical culture that is based on thinking outside

of the hospital, the ambulatory surgical center, or the magnetic reso-
nance imaging facility. It means recognizing that the patient's environmental context is important to consider as well as the need to support
periodic follow-up to make sure that people with chronic illnesses are
not subject to the risk of destabilizing.

One program is attempting to move away from medical supervi-
sion as much as responsible care culture will allow. A Stanford University School of Medicine initiative that started in the 1990s and that
is now making a concerted effort to scale up is entitled the Chronic
Diseases Self-Management Program. The essence of the program is
derived from teaching people with chronic diseases how to be in
charge of their own health.

> The Chronic Disease Self-Management Program is a workshop given
> two and a half hours, once a week, for six weeks, in community settings
> such as senior centers, churches, libraries and hospitals. People with dif-
> ferent chronic health problems attend together. Workshops are facili-
> tated by two trained leaders, one or both of whom are non-health
> professionals with a chronic diseases [sic] themselves.
>
> Subjects covered include: 1) techniques to deal with problems such
> as frustration, fatigue, pain and isolation. 2) appropriate exercise for
> maintaining and improving strength, flexibility, and endurance, 3)
> appropriate use of medications, 4) communicating effectively with
> family, friends, and health professionals, 5) nutrition, and 6) how to
> evaluate new treatments. (Stanford University School of Medicine,
> 2010)

The idea behind this California-based program is that people with
chronic illnesses have similar concerns and that they have to deal not
only with their diseases but also the impact on their lives and emo-
tions. The leadership is furnished by trained laypeople who deploy
coping strategies in the form of planning action and getting feedback,
problem-solving techniques, and decision-making training; this process is considered as important as the content that is transmitted
(Schneider, 2010). From the perspective of a person with several
chronic conditions, who reviewed a number of programs and
reviewed this book in manuscript form, this kind of peer support
appears to be outstanding.

The program in the three-year randomized control stages, completed in 1996, has been shown to offset the costs of medical care,
emergency department visits, as well as hospital admissions. Significant improvements in self-reported general health as well as mental
health were also found (Long et al., 2001).

Finally, I note with regret that despite these encouraging results of a chronic disease self-management program, now disseminated throughout the United States, and with training available on a fee-schedule basis, the relationship between medical home activities and costs are not well researched. According to a study of 35 practices using the medical home, the Commonwealth Fund authors (Zuckerman et al., 2009) found no evidence of additional costs associated with greater intensity of the presence of medical home activity in one practice versus another. This finding deserves a more drill-down approach since if you can get the same results with less intensive investments of time and effort, then the medical home model will be shown to be even more cost effective than it has been.

In this Commonwealth Fund review, wide variation in costs based on the use of information technology did exist, with higher use practices spending $11,000 per full-time equivalent physician compared with $8,000 spent in the average practice. The authors made no effort to determine other cost offsets for these 35 practices, as shown in other studies discussed in this chapter, and which could be a major incentive for adoption of the medical home model in integrated health care practices. Cost reduction remains uncertain in this age of health care reform, despite language in the Affordable Care Act to promote it in demonstration projects and scaled-up redesign of the delivery system. The authors of the bills that became the Affordable Care Act listened closely to advocates for massive expansion of primary care because it would lead to a reduction of the use of expensive medical interventions, a cause that goes back to the 1970s among health-care reformers, which spawned the training of nurse practitioners and physician assistants.

Not surprisingly, primary care professional associations have spearheaded the revival of primary care for people with chronic illnesses. Despite their enthusiastic endorsements of the medical home by professional associations that would benefit by it becoming a universal way of delivering primary care, there is concern among health policy experts that there is little information or systematic research on whether there is appropriate service utilization where the patient-centered medical home is the gold standard of care. It has been suggested by some thoughtful skeptics that the medical home model may keep some patients from getting subspecialty care when they absolutely need it as well as keeping some patients from unnecessary subspecialty care. The ghost of the "gatekeeper" from out of the early iterations of managed care that took hold in the last decade of the twentieth century, and the most tightly run health maintenance organizations of yesteryear, appears to be lurking behind this humanistic approach to medical care. Moreover, there is a trace of the fear that the use of a physician extender approach in the PCMH is a kind of second class primary care, even when multiple disease management is the goal of the provider team.

Furthermore, beyond these criticisms is the recognition by health policy analysts that there are "no direct incentives to other providers to work collaboratively with primary care providers in achieving" high-quality care at lower cost (Rittenhouse, Shortell, and Fisher, 2009). There is also the structural gap, a proverbial firewall, that exists between the doctors who save money by reducing hospital utilization and the lack of a mechanism for passing on some of the financial benefits of these savings to the patient with a chronic illness.

There are also a number of doubters in the health policy and service delivery fields who are not sure that the PCMH has proven to be a cost savings driver and can be scaled up so that it can work in many different clinical settings. While large practices have introduced this concept, we don't know how well it would work in medium- and small-sized practices. In addition, the pilot projects that have attempted to introduce PCMH have often left out some of the elements that the designers regard as essential, so that even when cost savings are generated, they may be based on a cut-down version of the full program. Finally, studies do not include the design costs (planning), and sometimes startup costs, when the results of care for people with chronic illnesses are compared with less integrated care (Sidorov, 2008). Yes, there are still some unanswered questions.

In particular, the disparity in how providers share financially is a particularly important issue to address and it concerns as well how expensive users of health care services because of functional limitations will be regarded as likely targets for cost reductions. Will they be avoided in favor of the selection of "the low hanging fruit"? It should be noted that along with rates of chronic illness that are associated with social class differences, there are also differences in the prevalence of disability in different populations. This presents a new challenge since the problems of how to deliver quality care that makes a difference in the lives of people with chronic illnesses, even when concerned about costs, must also confront the complexities driven by other concerns.

In answer to some of these criticisms, the previously mentioned patient-centered medical home demonstration, initiated by Seattle-based Group Health, attempted to deal with some of the complexities found in this new model of primary care (Reid et al., 2009). The prospective and quasi-experimental before and after evaluation undertaken with a random sample of patients, staff, and two control clinics sought to show better outcomes for patients with chronic illness at lower cost. Patients in the demonstration fared better when it came to their health care experiences than those in control clinics on six of the seven patient experience scales. Patients in the PCMH relied more on e-mail, phone, and specialist visits than did those in the control clinics but used fewer emergency services (Reid et al., 2009, p. e71). With 29 percent fewer emergency department visits, PCMH subjects helped the program save a substantial amount of money. Most importantly, the PCMH demonstration was able to change practice to encourage more access, longitudinal relationships, comprehensiveness, and coordination—all major features of quality primary care. As the authors state:

> In addition to system-wide improvements in quality, we found greater improvements in the composite measure of quality at the PCMH, indicating improvement across multiple conditions and clinical situations. (Reid et al., 2009, p. e79)

The authors make a great effort to show that this approach to care improvement is far superior to a disease-centered perspective because of the comprehensiveness and continuity of the services delivered, while conceding that there were limits to this study because it was an intervention at a single clinic and that survey responses varied widely from clinic to clinic.

The previous discussion of pilot projects was established to present these efforts as the result of the design work of the physicians and other providers who got them off the ground. A new national survey of patient-centered medical home demonstration projects (Bitton, Martin, and Landon, 2010, p. 584) gives the reader a cumulative view, showing that there are quite a number of projects around the country, even after eliminating those efforts that were nested in larger delivery systems rather than being truly independent start-ups. All told, the remaining numbers involved in the survey were impressive and made it appear that there is a solid basis for scaling up the patient-centered medical home. The study was based on a total of 26 robust demonstrations in 18 states; nearly five million patients received services from 14,000 physicians.

A large number of these pilot projects used the chronic care model (CCM) to develop the services required by their patients. As the authors state,

> The CCM identifies aspects of care systems that must be addressed to lead to significant improvements in chronic disease care. As applied to practice transformation, it provides guidance to practices on the types of initiatives they should undertake, working collaboratively with other practices within a learning collaborative. (Bitton, Martin, and Landon, 2010, p. 590)

The use of this model was supported financially mainly by a combination of traditional fee-for-service payments, per-person per-month fixed payments to support care coordination to help limit the quest for volume that has been criticized as one of the reasons primary care has deteriorated so much in the United States, and bonus payments for superior performance (Bitton, Martin, and Landon, 2010, p. 586). In none of the projects visited was there any effort to introduce bundled payments and partnerships with hospitals or medical centers to help keep patients from being admitted for inpatient care.

The surveyors were disappointed to see that the plans for evaluation of the impact of these pilot projects were not well developed. And while key informants at each project were interviewed, there were no attempts to interview patients regarding their opinions about the chronic-care model and whether it was an advance over previous efforts to assist them. Since the patient is supposed to be a partner in the chronic care model, this seems to be a serious design flaw.

In the next chapter I will review the problems and opportunities of people with disabilities who often have chronic conditions, and who also are concerned about their independence and want to be productive despite the often-defining statuses related to limiting conditions. Members of this segment of the chronic illness population have restrictions to their capacities to conduct activities of daily living and deficits in their ability to manage their lives as well. How PCMH would work with people with both disabilities *and* serious chronic illnesses is one of the vital topics addressed in Chapter 5.

# 5

# Disability and Chronic Illness

Accessing quality chronic care is a major frontier for people with disabilities to some extent because of the care system's bias toward acute care and making people well, rather than on optimizing a person's independence and productive capacities. People with disabilities spend a good deal of their lives combating chronic illness; they also do not live as long as people without disabilities. When people with intellectual disabilities continue to survive into later life, increasingly as a result of advances in health care so that congenital defects can be repaired and the impact of infections can be reduced to a minimum, there is still wonder expressed by clinicians when a person does *not* become a victim of common chronic disease associated with that particular intellectual disability. With no signs of clinical dementia, an individual with Down's syndrome in his 70s can become the subject of a published paper in a reviewed journal on successful aging (Krinsky-McHale et al., 2008). In contrast, conferences devoted to aging and intellectual disabilities, still known in some parts of the health world as developmental disabilities, will often present to parents and agency staff the symptoms to look out for in the aging person with an intellectual disability.

Early onset of Alzheimer's disease is often identified in adults with Down's syndrome, in part, a risk attributed to the over-expression of the amyloid precursor protein, found on chromosome 21, and the generator of a plaque that emerges during the fourth decade of life (Hof et al., 1995). In this case, the association found between dementia and Down's syndrome is genetic, while the higher risk for some common chronic diseases and disabilities does not have such a clear association.

It is often the case that people with disabilities, individuals with limitations in (1) activities of daily living, (2) limitation in instrumental activities of daily living, and (3) limitation in the performance of physical tasks, are also more likely than people without these limitations to be at significant risk for secondary conditions as well, a result of having a disability. Additionally, people with disabilities are also more likely than those without disabilities to have comorbidities, or health conditions that develop independently of the primary condition. Not being directly related to the primary condition, these comorbidities require vigilance in disease management, although with some behavioral disabilities the difficulty of the physical examination can limit the actual surveillance that takes place. I will attempt in this chapter to answer the following questions, based on the state of accumulated knowledge on the relationship between disability and chronic illness, as well as what kinds of care systems are most effective for dealing with a population at risk for serious chronic illness.

- What are the relevant characteristics of the disability population with regard to chronic illness?
- What are the consequences of being born with disabilities?
- Are there diseases that require chronic care that do not emerge among those born with disabilities until late in life?
- Under what conditions can behavioral health, also known as mental health treatment, be integrated with primary care?
- Based on these characteristics, how can we strategically target programs to reduce the health needs of this population?

To gather information about a wide range of behaviors and characteristics that affect the health of the American population, the Centers for Disease Control has undertaken a project for the past 20 years that has helped the states survey adults. Entitled the Behavioral Risk Factor Surveillance System or BRFSS, it has focused on behaviors and conditions that create health risks and that are linked with the leading causes of death such as heart disease, cancer, stroke, diabetes, and injury. The risk factors include lack of physical activity, being overweight, not using seat belts, and, not surprisingly, using tobacco and alcohol. In addition, there are several questions about whether the respondent received preventive medical care such as flu shots (e.g., H1N1), Pap smears, mammograms, and colorectal cancer screening.

Information is collected through telephone surveys conducted by the health departments of all 50 states plus the territories annually to determine high-priority health issues, detect emerging health issues, and identify populations at highest risk for illness, death, and disability through an analysis of data according to the respondents' age, sex, education, income, and race/ethnicity. The data are not simply collected because of academic interest in the causes and consequences of chronic diseases. Information is utilized to create preventive interventions, monitor effectiveness of these efforts, and support health-promoting community policies and programs. Note that the information on demographics can help target public health campaigns that support health promotion.

Monthly telephone interviews conducted with individuals ages 18 and older have led in the past to the total of 350,000 interviews a year, making the BRFSS the largest health survey conducted in the United States. One of the research questions that could be answered through the analysis of the data is whether people with disabilities were more likely than those adults without disabilities to have a chronic disease. In addition, are individuals with disabilities more likely than others to rate their health status differently when given a choice ranging from poor to excellent? Further along, does this rating lead to consequences regarding their perception of their independence and productivity when it comes to competing in the world of work?

Analysts at two state health departments—New York and Michigan—were able to answer these questions. The BRFSS contains two questions that help to identify adults with disabilities:

- Are you limited in any way in any activities because of physical, mental, or emotional problems?
- Do you have any health problem that requires you to use special equipment, such as a cane, a wheelchair, a special bed, or a special telephone?

Follow-up questions were triggered by "yes" answers to either screening question. Answers to these questions helped the analysts to determine whether disabilities were mild or severe. These questions related to whether the respondent needed the help of others with personal care needs, such as eating, bathing, or dressing (activities of daily living). In addition, several questions were asked about whether the help of others was needed in doing household chores, necessary business, shopping, and getting around for other purposes (instrumental activities of daily living).

According to the New York State BRFSS, people with disabilities were less likely than those without disabilities to meet recommended standards for physical activity. And those who required assistance in the activities of daily living and the instrumental activities of daily living, as mentioned in the previous paragraph, were half as likely to meet recommended physical activity requirements. When it comes to the risks of being overweight, again the individuals who required assistance with twice as likely as individuals without disabilities to be obese (Paeglow, 2007). Clearly there seems to be a connection between lack of physical activity and obesity, making the individual more vulnerable to such diseases as type 2 diabetes, although the direction of causality may not always be that lack of physical activity leads to obesity since obesity can also lead to inactivity.

Diseases are also more likely to be mentioned by respondents with disabilities than those without, and individuals who require assistance were far more likely to be diabetic or have a history of cardiovascular disease. Only 5 percent of adults with no disability had a history of cardiovascular disease compared with 27 percent of respondents who mentioned that they required assistance, with similar differences found when diabetes was the disease in question.

In the Michigan study, conducted in 2007, an estimated 23 percent in that state identified themselves as disabled according to the screening questions. The comparisons were shocking. In sum, "Those with disabilities were much more likely to be in fair to poor health compared with those without disabilities (41% to 7%) and less likely to be in good or excellent health (60% vs. 93%)." Beyond self-ratings, it is important to note that individuals with high risk of chronic disease are also more likely to require health services.

Even when people with disabilities are covered by Medicare, this social insurance program does not work as well for younger beneficiaries with disabilities than it does for older Americans. Medicare provides health insurance for eight million people with permanent disabilities who are eligible for Social Security Disability Insurance, or SSDI. There is a 29 month waiting period for Medicare once SSDI eligibility is established. There have been few attempts to find out how well Medicare works for people with permanent disabilities. We do know that during periods of economic downturns, more people apply for SSDI than during prosperous times since there are more barriers to employment that make people with disabilities less competitive with other potential hires without disabilities.

What is life like on SSDI, a full disability and income maintenance program? Juliette Cubanski and Patricia Neuman (2010) of the Kaiser Family Foundation used administrative data from the Center for Medicare and Medicaid Services to draw a sample of nonelderly disabled beneficiaries. Conducted in late 2008, the survey sampled 3,913, with 2,288 individuals with permanent disabilities between the ages of 18 and 64 and 1,625 people 65 years or older. The mailed survey was completed and returned by 39 percent of the younger and 47 percent of the older Medicare beneficiaries.

The population of interest to the Kaiser Family Foundation investigators faced multiple afflictions that Medicare beneficiary status did not fully mitigate. Among the younger permanently disabled, half reported having five or more chronic conditions, as compared to 25 percent of the elderly. Twice as many of the younger respondents reported feeling sad or depressed some or all of the time during the past year, and four times as many reported experiencing severe or very severe pain in the past month. The combination of both mental and physical ailments was greater among the nonelderly disabled than among the elderly Medicare recipients. Given the kinds of health problems they faced, it should come as no surprise that the young permanently disabled respondents reported higher use rates of hospitalizations and emergency department visits than did the older Medicare recipients.

Access to doctors and health care facilities, out-of-pocket costs, and transportation difficulties were clearly identified among the permanently disabled as persistent problems for them even with Medicare coverage. Those Medicare recipients with supplemental support from Medicaid, known as the dually eligible because of their low incomes, were better able to get care. Other sources of supplemental support that required payment were not nearly as effective and did not supply some of the other benefits found through Medicaid such as long-term and home and community-based care, programs often desired by people with disabilities and their families.

The disproportionate use of health services by people with disabilities transcends national borders and confirms the findings from the previously discussed studies in New York and Michigan, as well as the Kaiser Family Foundation study. A Canadian study, conducted in the province of Ontario, reviewed the hospitalization data for all persons with an intellectual disability, between 1995 and 2001 (Balogh, Hunter, and Quellette-Kuntz, 2005). The authors found that a substantial proportion of hospitalizations of this particular part of the population were for mental disorders (40%) such as schizophrenia and depression. As found south of the border, the Canadian study noted that there were frequent admissions for conditions that could have been managed (ambulatory-care sensitive) on an outpatient basis. This can be a high maintenance population, according to experiences in health care utilization recorded in the United States.

And because people with intellectual disability have a hard time cooperating with regular dentists, 4 out of 10 same-day surgery patients were admitted to hospital for dental procedures. Sometimes special care dentistry can prevent same-day surgery admissions for routine care but these kinds of clinics are not available in every community. In my experience with a community-based special care dentistry program, parents will give it a standing ovation when it is mentioned in public meetings associated with family care for people with developmental disabilities.

Special care dentistry is considered by some professionals in the field of intellectual disabilities as a vehicle for getting more than care of the mouth and teeth done. There is, on occasion, an attempt, promoted at developmental disability clinics, to do one-stop diagnosis and treatment on people who can be uncooperative. The idea is that when a patient with intellectual disabilities is under anesthesia, this is an opportunity to draw blood, check ears and clean out ear wax, and perform various tests. Parents tell me that it can be extraordinarily difficult to get these procedures arranged for and done because of scheduling conflicts and the limited window of opportunity available for add-ons to the dental work.

Often overlooked in discussions of disabilities and chronic care are the challenges generated by the presence of mental illness, a complication noted in the Canadian study. The intermittent, although sometimes persistent, nature of flare-ups among people with psychiatric histories makes them difficult to examine and treat in primary care settings. Depressions can last six months or more and clearly efforts to reduce their length can result in better health care as well as considerable savings to the health care payers (Pignone et al., 2002).

The neglect of physical conditions by this population, without primary-care interventions, means that the top 10 percent of patients account for 60–70 percent of health care utilization costs (Berk and Monheit, 2001). In most instances, repetitive hospitalizations are incidents that account for the overutilization and extra costs. Still, there are few primary care providers with the appropriate training and experience to care for people with disabilities; and even when a provider has skills and experience with one kind of disability, it does not mean the provider can transfer those skills to other people with different disabilities.

Efforts undertaken at the Martin Luther King Intensive Wellness Program to create continuity of primary care for a population with psychiatric histories were based on an interdisciplinary team that provided an advanced medical home. The kind of follow-up post-hospitalization with some of the patients with severe or poorly controlled diabetes reduced the number of hospital admissions while increasing dramatically the frequency of outpatient visits. The designers of this service admit the care will be expensive in this "advanced medical home" but no more so than what was not done in the past, which was also costly (Levine, 2009). With funding from foundations with missions devoted to changing the health care delivery system, e.g., the California Health Care Foundation, some model programs have emerged and have produced impressive outcomes. While there are new efforts underway to understand how we can do better with difficult and vulnerable populations, there has not been a scaling up of financing and planning-wise activities to deal with the full numbers of eligible patients for these programs. Patients with disabilities are part of the national experiment concerning how to deliver quality chronic care that can make a difference. We are just at the beginning of the formulation of a new paradigm on how to furnish care for populations that create challenges to integrating behavioral health and primary care.

Wellness is, according to experts, based usually on involvement in appropriate physical activities. People with disabilities who are also advocates have long noted that overweight and obesity is difficult to avoid without access to community athletic facilities and commercial fitness centers. And with obesity, if not overweight, all too often leading to diabetes, there is little attention paid to other secondary disabilities or chronic conditions. In the second decade of the twenty-first century, it is often noted that we live in an era characterized by an emergence of orthopedic problems that require knee or hip replacements.

Beyond the burdens of obesity, another challenge within our health care system is the disparities found through retrospective analysis when determining whether access to services is racially bound. In a South Carolina study of treatment via antiviral medication by a Medicaid population with an influenza diagnosis, while most patients had two or more comorbid chronic diseases, a basis for defining them as people with disabilities, white patients were far more likely to be treated than African American patients (Leon, McDonald, Moore, and Rust, 2009).

Racial disparities are often matched by the separation of people with severe disabilities from the community. Even people with disabilities who might need only a few hours of care may wind up in nursing facilities because care in the community could not be arranged. The Community Choice Act, folded in to various versions of health care reform in 2009 and supported strongly by the disability community, would pay for care at home, a new version of long-term care that would make a normal round of life possible for many people with disabilities and serious chronic illnesses.

It has also been established that supportive care services delivered at home can be less expensive than care delivered at nursing facilities. Community integration means that some of the overlay of expenditures related to institutionally based care can be peeled away. Moreover, care at home can reduce the dangers of becoming infected by viruses that spread rapidly in nursing facilities. Chris Hilderbrant (2009), the director of the Advocacy Center for Disability Rights, calls the Community Choice Act the vehicle for eliminating "the institutional bias that forces people into expensive facilities, rather than providing service at home."

Participation in community living may present its own struggles, particularly with regard to gaining access to expert health care. Access to providers with specialized knowledge that can assist a person with a particular disability may be difficult. If a person with a disability has public health insurance (i.e., Medicaid and Medicare), there may be fewer choices among doctors since some physicians will not see patients with Medicaid or Medicare coverage because of the low rates they pay for office visits. Paying out-of-pocket for medical care may be difficult for a person without an income beyond public assistance of one kind or another. Transportation to a doctor's office or a clinic may also be unaffordable for a person with a disability on a limited income. And medical offices and the examination equipment may not be accessible for people who use wheelchairs or have need of assistance getting in and out of a wheelchair.

The limits to medical care do not end when physical accessibility is established. People with hearing loss may also require American Sign Language interpreters or written materials. Additionally, some of the information that is available via electronic communication technology can create enormous barriers for people with disabilities so that such mundane tasks as finding a provider that is part of an insurance company's network can be incompatible with and therefore inaccessible to individuals who use screen readers, common devices that those who are blind use regularly. Learning how to use this assistive technology has become common during the last five decades in the United States, often the result of new opportunities in education for children with disabilities. The United States is catching up to other countries in terms of the availability of products that can help level the playing field or enhance communication and reduce physical barriers.

Assistive technology can be highly sophisticated and computer directed devices or it can be the kind of things, such as list making and check-off procedures, that have been used to prevent airlines from taking off with deficits in the mechanical and electrical parts of the planes, and which have been recently introduced into hospital practice to prevent the spread of infection.

Professionals who work with individuals who are cognitively challenged and who also are required to manage chronic illnesses call for simple devices that would allow adults with intellectual deficits to keep track of their health. The proliferation of these techniques can also assist elderly people with short-term memory deficits.

According to Terri McLaughlin (2010) at the Boston-based Federation for Children with Special Needs, the need for ways of guiding an adult with diabetes who is also cognitively challenged was met by the parents of a certain young man, who developed a simple eight-page booklet that fits in the pocket of his glucose meter. The idea is that the book can be utilized by staff at his school to help him avoid carbohydrates, even though he cannot "count carbs." Insulin dosages are also managed via this booklet so he can figure out how many units he needs to take given his carbohydrate intake. Again, a staff person will review his dosage of insulin before he takes it to make sure it is correct. McLaughlin suggests that there are not many ways that those with intellectual deficits can manage their chronic illnesses in the same way as in the case of the young Bostonian who was able to get help from the MASS GENERAL Diabetes Center and can stick to the right diet. (Readers can help create an inventory of this kind of assistive technology by responding directly to Ms. McLaughlin at tmclaugh@fcsn.org.) Managing chronic illness is also important to start during childhood, whether disability is in the picture or is not, as well as in our adult years.

Through a personal communication, McLaughlin (2010) suggests that the best way to get the "An everyday diabetes guide for Whitney" is through an e-mail message. She also notes that there are few resources or information available to help students with intellectual disabilities manage a chronic illness. Moreover, she advocates that this type of learning should start early so that students with chronic illness stay healthy and can enjoy life after high school; she recommends that this kind of guidance for self-advocacy and health management be part of the students transition plan.

## CHILDREN, DISABILITY, AND CHRONIC CARE

There has been a major revolution in the United States in the care and education of children born with disabilities in the past 50 years. The revolution started with the Education of All Handicapped Children Act, first passed in 1975 and since then lightly federally funded. This act, basically a civil rights law and now called the Individuals with Disabilities Education Act (IDEA), was reauthorized in 2002. These transformations in education have not been without enormous costs, both human and financial.

It is logical that a society that requires that all children go to school, despite the challenges that some bring to education, will also require that they have the assistance that they need to get through the school day. Some of this assistance is in the form of aides in the classroom and other kinds of assistance may mean functioning wheelchairs. If the system breaks down, as it did in Long Island, New York, then children cannot get to school, sit properly in the classroom, or do homework. A firm that sold and serviced wheelchairs ended that part of their appliance for people with handicapping conditions business because of declining reimbursement from Medicaid and Medicare. The appliance delivery system can be fragile and the concerns expressed by parents and consumers means that their chronic health needs, often dependent on these ways to maintain independence and inclusion, can be called into question (Whittle, 2009).

With the Great Recession advancing and state budgets running excessive deficits, even fiscally conservative states such as Kansas have had to rein in Medicaid expenditures because state revenues have not kept up with state expenses. Reimbursements to providers of durable medical equipment were sharply reduced in 2010 and businesses throughout the Jayhawk State were unwilling to operate at a loss to fulfill orders for Medicaid recipients, who clearly could not cross state lines to utilize their benefits (Hollingsworth, 2010).

The story of the loss of access in Bethpage, New York, to wheelchairs for children with mobility problems, and in Topeka, Kansas, as well, and in Medicaid budget cutbacks for their maintenance is a microcosm of the needs expressed by cohorts of children born prior to term. The lower the gestational age at birth, as identified in a study done in Norway of the premature and those born at full term, the greater the long-term prevalence of individuals who need assistance. The risk of being born with cerebral palsy was 900 times greater for infants born between 23 to 27 weeks of gestation, compared with those born at 37 weeks or later. Mental retardation or intellectual disability was 4.4 percent vs. 0.4 percent for children born between 23 and 27 weeks of gestation. And premature births were 10 times more likely than non-premature births to result in receiving a disability pension. For this cohort born between 1967 and 1983, the risks of medical and even some social disabilities (level of education attained) in adulthood increased with decreasing gestational age (Moster et al., 2008).

Birth may not be the beginning of the kinds of long-term care required but disability during childhood leads to increased therapy costs, home adaptations, and specialized day care. Families that start out poor may have greater difficulty managing with a child with a disability and families with a child with a disability may become poor as a result of extra expenses. The National Survey of America's Families, conducted in 2002 by two research and advocacy associations, the Urban Institute and Child Trends, discovered that among the 42,000 households reached, those families with a disabled child expressed greater worries that their food would run out, that food did not last, or that meals had to be skipped. In addition, the parents of a child with a disability were twice as likely as other parents to receive emergency funds or were unable to pay the rent (Parish et al., 2008).

The needs for services and the costs of care for a child with a serious chronic illness or disability are exacerbated when the two conditions are combined. In fact, the analysis of recent cross-sectional data derived from the 2005–2006 National Survey of Children with Special Health Care Needs (CSHCN) found that parents of children with neurologic conditions were more likely to report unmet health care needs for their child than other parents of CSHCN. Parents of CSHCN with at least two chronic conditions reported more visits for health care services, the need for more services, and more unmet needs than parents of CSHCN with a single condition (Bitsko et al., 2009, p. S343).

The co-occurrence for children of neurologic and other medical conditions poses a difficult problem in care coordination for this population. Primary care, mental health care, education, and specialized medical services are requirements that may be difficult to optimize in a service system that does not create financial incentives to furnish care coordination. The data analysis performed by Bitsko and her coauthors (2009) was able to identify conditions included in the *Diagnostic and Statistical Manual of Mental Disorders* (*DSM*) that strongly correlated with poor access to service and a disproportionate set of service needs. As they state:

Notably, the non-DSM-disorder subgroup was least likely to have unmet needs or to be dissatisfied with care coordination, whereas the 2 subgroups of CSHCN with multiple conditions had the greatest unmet needs and dissatisfaction with care coordination. Care coordination may be more challenging for children with multiple conditions, which could result in more unmet needs among this subgroup of CSHCN. (p. S349)

The origins of the patient-centered medical home (PCMH), as discussed in the previous chapter, were derived from primary care and specialty care pediatricians who had to deal with children with serious chronic illnesses and disabilities. While the PCMH has spilled over its boundaries and now is a major organizing concept when it comes to furnishing advanced primary care for aging patients, there is still a persistent interest in the model among faculty who participate in programs that train medical providers who will serve children with special health care needs. Some of the 37 Leadership Education in Neurodevelopmental Disabilities programs, or LENDs, have attempted to transfer medical home competencies to their trainees. In partnership with the American Academy of Pediatrics and the Association of University Centers on Disabilities, a program at the University of Utah headed by Judith Holt, PhD, has launched in 2009 a program whereby postdoctoral fellows receive additional training regarding their future roles as part of a team in medical homes (Holt, Esquivel, and Pariseau, 2010).

Guided by the view that medical care should be accessible, continuous, comprehensive, family-centered, and coordinated, trainees learn how to implement a specific care plan as part of an organized team. This approach builds on the LEND curriculum that fosters "interdisciplinary teamwork and service provision, family-centered care, cultural competency, and leadership in policy and advocacy" (Holt, Esquivel, and Pariseau, 2010, p. 2).

The objectives of the entire LEND program are formidable, including

- advancing the knowledge and skills of all child health professionals to improve health care delivery systems for children with developmental disabilities;
- providing high-quality interdisciplinary education that emphasizes the integration of services from state and local agencies and organizations, private providers, and communities;
- providing health professionals with skills that foster community-based partnerships; and

- promoting innovative practices to enhance cultural competency, family centered care and interdisciplinary partnerships. (Holt, Esquivel, and Pariseau, 2010, p. 4)

The LEND programs can help supply a greater capacity to care for children with special needs. However, how to pay for these services has not been a question that received resolution in our country. The need for systems change when it comes to financing is evident. While there are Children's Health Insurance programs in every state where parents can voluntarily purchase subsidized insurance for a child, there are still gaps in coverage for this population. The National Survey of Children with Special Health Care Needs, 2005–2006, found that almost 9 percent of the families surveyed said that the CSHCN had no insurance for at least part of the study year. Still, even among those with insurance, parents volunteered in one out of every three interviews that the insurance coverage was inadequate, given the child's condition, and one out of five families spent $1,000 or more out of pocket for medical expenses for the CSHCN. In particular, dental care for children who require anesthesia can run up annual out-of-pocket expenses. Almost as many parent respondents said the child's conditions caused financial problems for the family. All of this valuable information is available in the Chartbook 2005–2006 for this important national study (Health Resources and Services Administration, 2009).

It is especially difficult to establish this kind of promotion of access to a variety of services when the family or the child is uninsured. The uninsured, whether healthy or with one or more chronic conditions, receive less in the way of services than those with insurance. Bitsko and her colleagues (2009) report that

> Among CSHCN with neurologic conditions, those with 2 or more neurologic conditions (either at least 2 DSM conditions or 1 of each type) were more likely than CSHCN with a single DSM condition to have inadequate insurance, be uninsured, have public health insurance, and be living in poverty. (p. S348)

This discussion of how mental health and neurologic disorders can create complications in the delivery of health care and other services to children with special health care needs may also be the basis of a question about what kinds of barriers are confronted by service providers when attempting to look at what adults with similar kinds of constellations of disorders.

Recognition of these barriers and how to eliminate them is one of the platforms of health care reform. The Affordable Care Act attempts to create new incentives and opportunities to improve home and community based services (HCBS) funded through Medicaid. These incentives, when rolled out, will make it possible for individuals with disabilities to remain in the community, permitting them to gain access to attendant care services, supported by a new federal Medicaid matching rate. In addition, new funding and coordination guidelines will drive the articulation between medical and long-term care services for people with chronic diseases (Sebelius, 2010b). Clearly, attention is being paid through this omnibus legislation to people with complicated situations, including those with both physical deficits and a need for mental health services.

A change in attitude by primary care providers to people with intellectual disabilities arguably is worth advocating for, independent of health care reform. When a child with intellectual disabilities ages out of the pediatric care system, there is often a dearth of primary care providers willing to become a permanent source of care. One parent recounted that she took her son to a physician with a strong reputation for ethical care only to be rudely disappointed.

> John was due to go under general anesthesia for dental work, and a physical examination was required. I very much wanted to get someone to listen to his heart, because both his father and I have heart problems, and no one had actually gotten him to hold still long enough to really listen. This much-touted doctor told me, "I will sign anything saying he is healthy enough for anesthesia, but I won't risk injury to myself by going near him."

Alternatively, this mother writes that on another occasion, when her son refused to go into an examining room, a different doctor came out and did the examination in the waiting room, "all the while playing with him and engaging him." Given John's intolerance of testing, this doctor kept his medical work to a minimum and treated symptoms as best he could rather than drill down more deeply to find causes.

Clearly, some comorbidities require special consideration. Do the models of care that have been constructed for adult patients with these comorbidities address the issue of what kinds of mental health services are required for adults with multiple special health care needs, among them psychiatric interventions? Are there ways of educating medical students about the extensive problems faced by families when they encounter members of the medical professions and  their reluctance to be responsible caregivers for people with intellectual disabilities? In the next chapter, I will try to address the first question, which focuses on the chronic care model. However, let me point out that there is already attention being paid to the writing of the regulations and rules associated with the Affordable Care Act and there are sharp eyes out there in the disability community.

When new rules and regulations are written, they sometimes weaken the intent of the legislation or fail to carry forward existing arrangements that work effectively. There are often lobbyists who seek to water down the responsibilities of the businesses and industries they represent so that they do not have to comply with the intent of the legislation. Laws such as the Affordable Care Act are only effective if they are implemented through regulations that include protections for patients with disabilities and chronic conditions so that they can access the care they need. The Consortium for Citizens with Disabilities (CCD), responding in the summer of 2010 to the Secretary of the Department of Health and Human Services (HHS), proposed final rules so that consumers are protected when they purchase a health plan that requires going through a primary care "gatekeeper." Often these plans come with the least expensive premiums and copays. The consortium recommended that people with disabilities and chronic conditions who know their condition well

> be given direct access to specialists because it . . . is efficient, less costly to the plan, and leads to better, more timely care. It is for these reasons that CCD believes the HHS Secretary should permit enrollees with disabilities and chronic conditions to select a willing specialist to serve as a case manager or primary care "gatekeeper" in plans that employ this delivery model. (CCD Health Task Force, 2010, p. 4)

Clearly, experience with this population suggests that the health maintenance organization (HMO) model, one option that will be available through state health insurance exchanges, may not be appropriate for people with multiple conditions. It is often the case that primary-care providers have limited experience with people with disabilities and chronic illnesses because they are seen infrequently in their practices. Perhaps within the HMO, it is possible to designate one primary-care provider as the generalist who becomes the onsite "specialist" in dealing with the requirements of people with disabilities and chronic illnesses so that changes in their condition will not be overlooked and speedy access to specialists will occur so that signs of deterioration can be identified and nipped in the bud through appropriate medical intervention.

The consortium also sought in August 2010 to remind the rulemakers at HHS that there should be no allowance of a reduction of benefits in existing health plans for what is covered or be less generous with services by establishing more restrictions on the number of visits for rehabilitation services, services extremely important to people with disabilities who are trying to maintain their level of functioning. Existing plans that will be "grandfathered" in under the Affordable Care Act, according to CCD, should not see any reduction in benefits or change in the structure of the plan, e.g., requiring prior authorization via a primary care physician where no authorization was previously required, or going from both in-network and out-of-network access to a closed panel of physicians. Similar warnings about changes in drug benefits were also issued in the letter from the CCD Health Task Force. These are challenges that affect the delivery of chronic care according to models that emerged from the advocates in Seattle during the past two decades, including more than one million subjects in studies of outcomes (Grumbach and Grundy, 2010).

Despite the CCD's concerns about losing out on benefits, there is substantial evidence from prospective and controlled studies that patient-centered primary care does create primary care that produces integrated delivery systems, including both private and public payers.

> investing in primary care patient centered medical homes results in improved quality of care and patient experiences, and reductions in expensive hospital and emergency department utilization. (Grumbach and Grundy, 2010, p. 1)

# 6

# The Chronic Care Model: Designed to Avoid the Avoidable

Sometimes a family story in a scholarly work is appropriate. I once had a plumber come to repair a leaky pipe in my basement and before he went ahead and tackled the obvious problem, he said, "Where shall I begin?" In other words, it was not just one leaky copper water pipe that had to be fixed, but so long as he was down there in my 75-year-old house, where probably a good deal of the plumbing was done by the Lithuanian seaman who jumped ship in New York Harbor and eventually started buying houses and fixing them up in the 1960s, there were many problems that were about to emerge. Could that have been a harbinger of a fateful future for this observer of the U.S. health care scene?

There are many coming crises in an old plumbing system if we don't start doing preventive maintenance now. The same thing can be said about the way chronic illness is addressed in the United States in the beginning of the second decade of the twenty-first century. Our work is cut out for us because there are structural hurdles to overcome to create a system of care that will keep people well, allow them to have a decent quality of life, and reduce the cost of health care (bending the curve) for the entire country by keeping people out of hospital beds and emergency departments. During the past decade, many small hospitals were closed, and even in larger locations, the number of beds available was reduced. Payers, both private and public, wanted to rein in health care costs and this target seemed to be obvious to health policy experts.

The Medicare payment system is a good place to start when it comes to driving spending down. First, hospitals were going to be penalized financially for admitting patients unnecessarily. Then the inpatient stay for Medicare patients was subject to limitations by additional financial penalties via the establishment and application of diagnostic review groups, with their average length of stay for particular organ systems and procedures. Incentives were created to keep beneficiaries out of the hospital by making primary care and specialty care more accessible in the community. This process to divert patients from hospital admissions and lengthy stays was so successful that physicians, sometimes with the assistance of hospitals and academic medical centers, created new locations to treat patients.

The nationwide effort at establishing greater access in the community for care for chronic illnesses was now evident when additional utilization data were reviewed. Specialty care was bending the cost curve—but in the wrong direction. It became obvious as to what had happened that, in 2009, Congress was willing to cut payments to physicians by about 20 percent to reduce Medicare expenditures. Even with reductions in the use of hospital care, chronic care costs in the community for Medicare eligible people has helped to fuel the rise in spending in that program. The cost of health care for the Medicare population continues to increase as the pattern of spending from 1997 to 2006 has shifted so that "medical conditions other than heart disease—diabetes, arthritis, hyperlipidemia, kidney disease, hypertension and mental disorders—accounted for more than a third in the rise in Medicare spending" (Thorpe, Ogden, and Galactionova, 2010, p. 2).

While some of the increased spending results from higher incidence of actual disease, such as diabetes, rather than better screening and diagnosis, the intensity of treatment via frequent office visits accounts for a large share of the growth in spending. Comparisons of the location of care for Medicare eligible individuals in the 1987 National Medical Expenditure Survey (NMES) and the 1997 and 2006 Medical Expenditure Survey (MEPS) found "Physician office visits rose to 21 percent of overall spending and more than tripled as a percentage of top-ten conditions spending. The percentage of spending for physician visits nearly doubled for heart disease and quadrupled for cancer" (Thorpe, Ogden, and Galactionova, 2010, p. 722).

Medicaid expenditures continue to increase annually, even with new payment structures in place. Clearly, the hospital-based medical model has shifted to the doctor's office, where multiple providers in various settings furnish episodic care to chronically ill patients, with more than half being treated for five or more chronic conditions annually. Typically, Medicare beneficiaries see two primary care physicians and five specialists, practicing in four different ambulatory care settings. Health care delivery is driven by financing and the holes in the system, mainly related to care coordination, cannot be filled without a change in how health care is paid for. Fee-for-service medicine hardly encourages coordination because a provider may lose out if the care was coordinated and remuneration was bundled (Pham et al., 2007).

We can all start out with a good idea of what patient-centered care is all about and that it is the direct opposite of the medical model, with its emphasis on organ systems and disease. Starting to see the whole human being, what the medical culture calls "the patient," is a paradigm shift in health care delivery. Breaking with the past, particularly the experiences of overworked house staff who would identify a patient by the disease he or she had when discussing treatment planning with colleagues, some physicians, starting in the 1970s, began seeing patients as "larger than the sum of their admissions" (Seifter, 2010, p. 21). Despite the growing humanistic approach to patients with chronic illnesses, we learned in the past chapters that the problem of how to deliver chronic care via a patient-centered medical home is not a simple one. It is also organizationally in competition with the industrial-strength model of disease management, a way of looking at the patient even more as a serviceable object. But there are some reasons to be hopeful based on the enormous power of the chronic care movement within health care when it comes to showing consumers that things do not have to be done in ways that only create profits for either hospitals or the disease management corporations that have sprung up so that the most difficult cases get stripped out or carved out of managed care because the needs for services in the community are so great.

The critical facts about chronic illness in America produce a call to action. The concern about patient-centered care has found its way into the Affordable Care Act that was signed into law by President Obama on March 23, 2010, a moment in legislative history in the United States that closely parallels the introduction of Medicare and Medicaid in 1965. An impressive amount of funding—$600 million—will be made available through appropriations associated with the new law to support a Patient Centered Health Research Center, which will fund pilot projects and demonstrations that will discover the effectiveness of the medical home and the chronic care model. Equally important, this center will help doctors understand and pass that understanding on to their patients that more care, especially invasive care, does not mean better outcomes (Leonhardt, 2010b). There is still far to go in getting the medical profession to admit that less is more and it will not come about right away. There is a shared belief among patients and providers that there is always something available in the medical armamentarium that will substantially prolong life and is better than palliative care. However, quality care often means that the primary-care provider takes time to explain what chronic illness is such as congestive heart failure and how best it can be managed. In turn, the physician also needs to take the time to learn from the patient his or her personal concerns in dealing with chronic illnesses.

There is also one major technological advance in information systems, requiring a national or statewide partnership, which can make chronic care more effective. Guiding the care of people with chronic illnesses are new methods of tracking who gets what treatment, particularly for people with rare conditions. Titled registries, these electronic data collection tools permit clinicians and researchers to identify the treatments used, the results obtained, and the health status of patients. These elements are the foundations for the widespread establishment of evidence-based practice. The average life expectancy, for example, of people with cystic fibrosis has been doubled for the estimated 30,000 people alive today in the United States with this life-threatening condition (Freudenheim, 2009, p. D1). There are also uses of this kind of data collection to determine how services can be improved and what additional conditions require interventions. When this method of data collection and monitoring of care was emulated by the National Parkinson's Disease Foundation, the early data showed that there was a wide variation in the treatments utilized and patients were often subject to additional diseases and cognitive deficits.

When there is decisive evidence regarding what works, registries have been shown to reduce death rates in cases of recurrent heart attacks and halve the annual death rate from HIV/AIDS (Freudenheim, 2009, p. D6). Going back to the beginning of the twenty-first century, diabetes registries have also been created to stratify patients according to risks, cue them when they need to take medication or prompt people to do urine analysis, as well as establish scores for physicians regarding their performances as caregivers (Bodenheimer, Wagner, and Grumbach, 2002a, p. 1778).

These data systems and alerts can be important in an aging society. Diabetes care is receiving a great deal of attention lately not just because of increased incidence (new cases) and prevalence (all cases existing at a single point in time) but because the costs of the disease, including treatment, pre-disease treatment, and lost productivity due to absence from work, has increased enormously. Students of the economic burdens of all forms of the disease seek to determine the costs by examining the savings in expenditures that would occur in the absence of diabetes or pre-diabetes (Dall et al., 2010). This estimation does not stop with medical expenditures but also includes the costs of lost productivity at the workplace.

As Dall and his colleagues (2010) point out, "One-fourth of U.S. adults have pre-diabetes and are at high risk for developing diabetes. By age sixty, approximately one in five U.S. adults has diabetes, and two in five have pre-diabetes" (p. 301). The financial burden in 2007 of the disease and its consequences exceeded $218 billion. While the collective costs of this disease may be shared through insurance premiums and Medicare and Medicaid payments, individuals with diabetes also pay disproportionately because of the trends in insurance coverage to have deductibles and copayments in employer-based insurance policies. And it is often the case that diabetes is accompanied by comorbidities that need treatment as well. The shifting of costs to the consumer of care clearly is an attempt to save money for employers, but it creates heavy financial burdens as well as emotional stresses for people with serious chronic illnesses.

Diabetes is not the only basis of costly treatment. The combination of diabetes and depression makes patient compliance less likely and therefore increases the likelihood that depressed individuals treated will have poorer outcomes than those where this serious and common mental disorder is not present (Ciechanowksi, Katon, and Russo, 2000). Similar findings were revealed when patients with a combination of depression and heart disease were followed prospectively (Jiang, Krishnan, and O'Connor, 2002). J. John Mann (2005), in his review article on the medical management of depression, also mentions that the treatment of epilepsy for a person with depression has poor results. Linkages between one or more chronic conditions, then, makes health services delivery experts attempt to come up with innovative strategies to do chronic care management under difficult circumstances. And part of the promise of these strategies is a reduction of costs in service delivery as well as patients being able to better self-manage their conditions. Visions of reduced spending in a system of health care where costs are unsustainable can be extremely exciting to those who are attempting to rein in expenditures.

## PATIENTS WITH MULTIPLE DIAGNOSES

It should come as no surprise that health policy analysts who are seeking to "bend the curve" in the growth of expenditures for chronic care (in the right direction) are most concerned about the spending that has gone on in the 15-year period between 1987 and 2002 for Medicare recipients with five or more chronic conditions. The costs of care have risen astronomically from 52 percent of Medicare spending to 76 percent (Bodenheimer and Berry-Millett, 2009, p. 1) and constitutes a red alert to experts interested in a health care industry that does not eat up every aspect of the gross domestic product. Even members of the angry Tea Party faction of the Republican Party might put aside their fantasies of "death panels" making end-of-life decisions to wonder whether something cannot be done about how to rein in these out-of-control costs. Anarchy in the medical marketplace cannot be permitted to continue if we are to establish a society that gets value from health care expenditures.

The future increase in the number of people becoming eligible for Medicare coverage as a result of the coming eligibility of the Baby Boom generation will also make care management for people with multiple chronic illnesses a great concern for any responsible citizens who want to see the costs of furnishing chronic care rise less precipitously than they have in the past decade and the quality of life of those who need chronic care management improve. Bodenheimer and Berry-Millet (2009) carefully define care management so that the focus is primarily on the patients who have multiple diseases.

> Care management is a set of activities designed to assist patients and their support systems in managing medical conditions and related psychosocial problems more effectively, with the aim of improving patients' health status and reducing the need for medical services. (p. 4)

How did this concept of care management come into being, given the pervasiveness of the medical model of care? Where did we get the idea that less medical care is more valuable than more care? A brief history is in order of how these ideas evolved. Thomas Bodenheimer, in all of his articles and published papers on primary care and the chronic care model, credits Ed Wagner and his associates for developing the model for the delivery of primary care to people with multiple chronic illnesses (Bodenheimer and Berry-Millet, 2009, p. 4; Bodenheimer, Wagner, and Grumbach, 2002a, p. 1775). Comorbidities, once again, seem to be the rule rather than the exception for patients with chronic conditions, according to research conducted at Johns Hopkins University, using data sets derived from claims information for nonelderly patients enrolled in a midwestern Blue Cross Blue Shield Point-of-Service managed care plan (Starfield, Lemke, Bernhardt, Foldess, Forrest, and Weiner, 2003). Resource utilization depended, according to the authors, on the degree of comorbidity rather than the diagnosis. This is a new and useful way to look at chronic care.

Another careful analysis done around the same time as the previously discussed article was based on comparing the 39 studies of chronic care interventions that used components of the new model of chronic care intervention as an experiment and where there was a control group to use as a basis for comparison so that it could be determined that there were positive outcomes and processes that resulted from the new way of delivering chronic care services. Bodenheimer, Wagner, and Gumbach (2002b) examined research evidence and identified components of the chronic care model that were consistently present in all patient-care demonstrations and used to assist patients with diabetes mellitus. These components were extracted from the work of Cochrane Review observers, an international team of experts in comparative effectiveness research, and comprised of physicians and health delivery system researchers who focused on randomized control studies and controlled before-and-after studies that mainly included subjects who were patients with diabetes. The Cochrane Review has been the gold standard in rigorous effectiveness studies for several decades. The four components of the chronic care model that were identified from the careful reviews of these studies were the following:

- **self-management support**, which usually involves Registered Nurses who are trained to teach patients and families the skills required to make early notice of declining health or worsening symptoms that can be responded to before going to the emergency department or being admitted to a hospital (Bodenheimer and Berry-Millett, 2009, p. 26)
- **decision support via educational materials and meetings for physicians**, including an assessment of patient needs, developing a care plan with the patient, family, and physician (Bodenheimer and Berry-Millett, 2009, p. 26)
- **delivery system design by introducing the use of case managers**, multidisciplinary teams, the training of RNs or advanced practice nurses to work with patients with multiple diagnoses, *and the scheduling of planned (diabetes) follow-up visits* (Bodenheimer and Berry-Millett, 2009, p. 26)
- **a clinical information system**, with reminders and feedback on physician performance (Bodenheimer and Berry-Millett, 2009, p. 32)

The selection of diabetes for these adventures in the reinvention of chronic care services is clearly the result of the goal of attempting to reduce costs by limiting hospitalizations and visits to the emergency departments of medical centers as well as seeking to combat seriously the comorbidities associated with this disease related to the circulatory system.

Similarly, there is a strong desire on the part of the remakers of chronic care to focus on the elderly with heart failure. Using a three-month advanced-practice nursing intervention for 239 patients who were ages 65 and older and hospitalized with heart failure, the team at the University of Pennsylvania Medical Center and various community hospitals in Philadelphia sought to reduce the number of rehospitalizations and expand the time until death of these chronically ill patients (Naylor et al., 2004, p. 675). The focus of the intervention by advanced practice nurses (APN), who used to be called nurse practitioners, was on preparation for discharge through planning and the development of a home follow-up protocol. This demonstration project took on older people with the chronic disease that results in the highest rates of readmissions to hospitals of any adult disease. This nuanced approach deserves a lengthy quote regarding what was done to change chronic care.

> The intervention included ... (1) a standardized orientation and training program guided by a multidisciplinary team of heart failure experts ... to prepare APNs to address the unique needs of older adults and their caregivers throughout an acute episode of heart failure; (2) use of care management strategies foundational to the Quality-Cost Model of APN Transitional Care, including identification of patients' and caregivers' goals, individualized plans of care developed and implemented by APNs in collaboration with patients' physicians, educational and behavioral strategies to address patients' and caregivers' learning needs, continuity of care and care coordination across settings, and the use of expert nurses to deliver and manage clinical services to high risk patient groups; and (3) APN implementation of an evidence-based protocol, guided by national heart failure guidelines. (Naylor et al., 2004, pp. 676–677)

The protocol was triggered by an initial APN visit within the first 24 hours of hospitalization. Daily visits during hospitalization took place, along with eight visits at home, including the first one within the first 24 hours of discharge. Phone contact also took place, and frequent visits were made during the first month, with a decreasing number of visits during the second and third month following discharge (Naylor et al., 2004, p. 677).

A randomized control trial took place, with a sample of 118 in the intervention and 121 in the control group and the results were some-what impressive but not all that was wished for. The time to the first readmission or death was longer for the intervention patients and at 52 weeks intervention group patients had fewer readmissions; mean total costs for the intervention group were $7,636 and $12,481 for the control group. Higher direct costs for visits by the APNs were offset by fewer visits to physicians, emergency departments, and readmissions. While there was evidence of improvements in the quality of life of patients who received the advanced practice nursing services, there were only short-term improvements demonstrated, as well as limited improvements in the physical dimension of living. Similarly, patient satisfaction was better in the intervention group at two and six weeks, but these differences did not continue in the long run (Naylor et al., 2004, p. 675).

This controlled study was a landmark because it was the first to show "reductions in re-hospitalizations caused by co-morbid conditions and reductions in overall hospitalizations and cost of elderly patients hospitalized with both systolic and diastolic heart failure" (Naylor et al, 2004, p. 683). With patients in the study averaging six comorbidities, APNs were guided by a flexible protocol that permitted them to attend to conditions that, if exacerbated, could result in readmissions, a distinct improvement over previous interventions with patients with heart failure that did not prevent readmissions for other causes. This holistic approach described by the reporters of this use of APNs also was supported by continuity in the care furnished by the same APN who saw the patient in the hospital, coordinated the discharge plan, and actualized it in the patient's home. The positive results of this kind of intensive transitional care of older adults hospitalized by a progressive condition, heart failure, have hardly been emulated in managed-care plans funded by commercial insurance or in Medicare Advantage plans.

## CHRONIC CARE MANAGEMENT AND DISEASE MANAGEMENT

The kind of transition management that Naylor and her associates undertook was complex to meet the needs of people with heart failure. Chronic care management for patients with complex medical needs is distinguished by advocates from the disease management approach, mentioned briefly earlier, and found in health plans that carve out care for patients with a particular condition and specializes in dealing with that disease and that disease only. This approach seeks to limit the amount of time and effort that a managed care plan spends with a patient and permits disease-management companies to focus exclusively on patients with one condition. These for-profit disease management companies do "cherry pick" and may avoid taking on patients with multiple diagnoses. Since they skim the cream they don't deal with the recondite cases that commend much attention. And naturally, as "one-trick ponies," the disease-management companies make true believers and missionaries for chronic care management uncomfortable.

Most importantly, the confrontation of multiple morbidities often makes the "road maps" for chronic care available through clinical practice guidelines inappropriate. To some extent the limited knowledge available is a result of the design of the research that drives the development of the guidelines. One of the great challenges faced when changing the health care system to focus on chronic care is that the knowledge base available through rigorous experimental and control group design means that people with several chronic illnesses are not considered appropriate subjects for these clinical research projects. More than 90 percent of individuals with diabetes have one or more comorbid conditions. It was only in 2009 through allocations in the economic stimulus package, also known as the American Recovery and Reinvestment Act (ARRA), were made available for effectiveness research. These funds, designed to jump-start the economy, also made possible the study of how to deliver more valuable services to people with multiple chronic conditions. This $20 million item includes an allocation of $12 million for the establishment of infrastructure development so that investigators can share data sets.

There are some powerful barriers that the profession of medicine and the organization of health service delivery have put up to keep the study of how to best care for people with multiple chronic illnesses. Parekh and Barton (2010) note the paradox that exists in health care research today that impedes a transformation to a multiple condition approach.

> The tremendous efforts in the fight against chronic disease have inadvertently created individual disease "silos," which are reinforced by specialty organizations, advocacy groups, disease management organizations, and government at all levels. (p. 1304)

There are still some basic guidelines available to quality care delivery, even without evidence-based practice. Care managers need to use the knowledge they derive from working with patients and their families to help them select patients who would benefit the most from care management. In doing so, they have to weigh the risks and benefits of putting that household into the program and whether or not the patient and the family are capable of learning the knowledge, acquiring the ability, and possessing the motivation to internalize what is needed to manage several diseases at once as well as handle several medications, with some having the potential for adverse interactions.

The amount of time that the patient at home is required to pay attention to symptoms that may indicate a worsening of a condition is extended over many months, and in some cases may be several years. Transferring the knowledge and ability that can allow patients to respond decisively to changes in their health status so that they can remain in the community may depend on excellent teaching or coaching by well-trained care managers and also on the selection of patients who are capable of picking up what is essential to do in the task of self-management of their chronic conditions.

Care management teams also need to establish the mechanisms for tracking patients over time to make sure that the steps required for self-management are undertaken. Moreover, self-management, as part of the care plan, may be subject to alterations when the household composition changes or when patients return to employment or other full-time activities. Revising the procedures during the course of care delivery is a form of continuous quality improvement that can save lives, eliminate unnecessary emergency room visits, and permit avoidance of hospitalizations.

These revisions to create a greater fit with patients may be absolutely necessary when dealing with the application of the chronic care model to the population past 80 years of age. David B. Reuben, MD, in writing about medical care for the final years of life, opines that there is little in the way of evidence to guide the care of patients with multiple morbidities because

> [o]lder individuals and those with co-morbidities are often excluded
> from clinical trials, and some conditions are difficult to study or have
> not received priority for research. Consequently, treatment recommen-
> dations often must extrapolate beyond the evidence base. (Reuben,
> 2009, p. 2687)

The employment of the elements of the chronic care model still requires the presence of a physician who is considered a primary-care provider, one who has the incentives to create and preserve the patient-centered medical home. This limited practice situation is compounded by trends in the selection of specializations as the careers of choice among recent medical school graduates. Medical school education and population requirements seem to be moving in opposite directions. While medical care is becoming more fragmented by the avoidance of primary care by recent medical school graduates because the potential income is too low to allow for the substantial payments due on medical student loans and the effort to maintain an upper-middle-class lifestyle, and a payment system that refuses to align incentives between hospitals and physicians, the need for person-centered chronic care management is more and more evident. The leaders of the charge for the preservation of the fee-for-service system, providers of specialty care and patients who did not want primary care providers authorizing visits to those specialists (as found in traditional health maintenance organizations), have not yet come up against the realities of twenty-first-century health care, wherein the blessings of medicine have created the enormous number of elderly people with multiple chronic comorbidities, and with each condition demanding attention at the same time.

The chronic care model, cautiously but consistently applied, may help to offset use of what has fast become yet another major expense for Medicare—the long-term care hospital that treats chronically ill patients, often fragile patients with multiple conditions. The model may also encourage greater continuity and coordination of care in the community, perhaps helping to limit the increase of what were originally called "step-down facilities" when they were first established in the 1980s.

In the past 25 years, more than 400 long-term acute care hospitals have opened in the United States, often encouraged by the fact that Medicare rates are higher for hospitals that treat patients with multiple conditions for a mean average of 25 days or more. Many of these hospitals are owned by for-profit companies and medical staffing is limited to doctors on call rather than being present at the facility (Berenson, 2010a, p. A1).

Patients in long-term care hospitals, while stable, are very sick, often require dialysis or ventilators, and may also have wounds that are taking a long time to heal. Long-term acute care hospitals are incentivized to keep patients in these facilities rather than return them to regular hospitals because Medicare will not pay multiple reimbursements if the time periods between stays at regular hospitals are brief. Still, Medicare, according to a lengthy investigation reported in the *New York Times* in 2010, has not addressed the problem of how to evaluate the quality of care being delivered by these relatively new kinds of programs. Alex Berenson, the author of this piece on our health care system via investigative journalism, also reported that there is a disproportionately higher rate of complaints from patients and their families at long-term acute care hospitals when compared to consumers at regular hospitals (Berenson, 2010b, p. A14). The conclusion may be drawn that care may be compromised in these long-term acute care facilities in order to limit expenditures. Yet for many patients with multiple life-threatening conditions, preparation for living in the community and taking charge of care through self-management actions brings the patient into a strategic position, going some distance beyond the patient-centered medical home, or as it is now called in some circles where innovation is ongoing, advanced primary care.

## BEYOND PATIENT CENTEREDNESS

In most of the discussions of the patient-centered medical home, found in Chapter 5, the patient is a partner in the care that is delivered rather than the orchestrator of that care. Some creative forces in the world of chronic care have attempted to shift the command structure of care to the patients themselves. The patient is arguably engaging in self-management, which includes "self-monitoring, environmental restructuring, getting support from family and friends, cognitive restructuring, and the relaxation response" (Cleland and Ekman, 2010, p. 1383). Empowerment for the person with a long-term condition means greater control over one's own life, a powerful concept that was at the beginning of the new culture—built around the ties between the personal and the political of the 1960s.

If individuals can gain command over how they live and work, then it follows that we need to free patients from the confines of taking orders from health-care personnel, even those who adhere to the patient-centered medical home philosophy. Shouldn't this approach have some desirable outcome such as reduced mortality rates? We can also anticipate that where customer productivity is involved, along with family and friends, this could generate savings related to the cost of delivery.

In one randomized trial, there was evidence suggesting that a chronic disease management program can improve health status while reducing hospitalization (Lorig et al., 1999). Self-management for a group of patients with heterogeneous chronic illnesses, including some with comorbidities, consisted of improvements in increased weekly minutes of exercise, cognitive symptom management, communication with physicians, self-reported health, health distress, fatigue, disability, and social role limitations. The comparison group was comprised of patients who were wait-listed for these services. The experimental group at six months into the study also had fewer hospitalizations and fewer days in the hospital. These hopeful findings encouraged other research studies to use the self-management counseling approach to patients with other diseases such as heart failure to encourage greater patient adherence to medical advice. Involved in the study conducted between 2001 and 2004 were 902 patients with mild to moderate heart failure and reduced or preserved systolic function.

A single center multiple hospital trial was conducted in the Chicago metropolitan area to determine the advantage of self-management counseling and heart failure education compared with health failure education alone (Powell et al., 2010). Patients who were randomized into the self-management group were given tip-sheets or guides and were taught self-management skills to implement the advice while patients in the control group received the same tip sheets but were called by phone to check on comprehension.

The emphasis in the treatment or experimental groups of 10 patients, which had 18 two-hour meetings, was on problem solving when patients identified barriers to implementing the tips received; patients then used self-management skills to overcome them. Treatment groups were led by health professionals with skills in conducting groups and a capacity to follow the protocol. The main outcome measure was death or heart failure during a median of 2.56 years of follow-up. The results were disappointing since the self-management counseling did not reduce heart failure–related deaths or hospitalization compared to the education intervention alone (Powell et al., 2010).

Perhaps the critical question to consider in this discussion of self-management is whether it can take place at a natural point in the life cycle when a child with a special health care need must undergo a transition from general pediatric and specialty care to adult medicine. In seeking uninterrupted, comprehensive, and accessible care, the planners of the transition are compelled to find an appropriate medical home with the assistance of a nurse or a care coordinator. Whoever becomes in charge of the medical home, be it a primary care physician or a subspecialist, their adolescent patient needs to acquire the knowledge, ability, and motivation to be a patient in the world of adult medicine. This may require a great deal of preparation via learning and role playing for the transition to take place; these activities might start several years before the actual hand-off takes place along with a search for adult subspecialists who can work with patients making the transition (White, 2009).

While many youths with serious chronic illnesses and disabilities are capable of self-management of their own health care, there is no guarantee that it will happen without effort to construct a medical home in a new setting for the patient. Consensus is emerging between various primary care provider associations, including the American Academy of Pediatrics and the American Academy of Family Physicians, and the American College of Physicians-American Society of Internal Medicine, that transition is a task for which participating providers need to be accountable.

> Coordination of care is a cornerstone of the medical home and an essential component of successful transition. There is much to be done if we are to make the transition from pediatric to adult health care a seamless one. The challenge to all health care providers is to promote self-determination in patients with SHCN and to prepare them with the knowledge and skills necessary to successfully navigate the adult system of care. Collaboration with colleagues who provide health care to adults is essential to improve the system of care. (White, 2009, p. 7)

Thus, there appears to be a continuum of reinvention in chronic care, from the most modest kinds of changes to the more adventurous efforts (just described) to empower patients so they can manage their own care, much like patients in the hospital can turn the dose of painkiller, usually morphine, up or down through an intravenous line. The patient as the "serviceable object," according to that great observer of human organizations, Erving Goffman, may be hard to find in the new era of delivery system as well as financing reform. As consumers, patients dread their financial *responsibilities* following a long hospital stay. Remaking chronic care is not only vital to create value in the delivery system but to make consumers feel less desperate about their chances of plunging into medical indebtedness. As we will see in the next chapter, financing often limits access to chronic care and makes consumers pay substantially through copays and deductibles when they need to receive assistance for multiple chronic conditions.

# 7

# Financing Chronic Care

Our health care system is out of alignment, as noted in the previous chapter when I wrote about the financial disincentives to promote medical homes and ambulatory care for people with chronic illnesses. Like anything out of alignment, such as wheels and tires, it runs inefficiently and needs to be corrected. The health care system is expensive and has grown approximately 2.8 percent faster annually than the rest of the economy and threatens to account for 30 percent of the gross domestic product in the year 2038. Many of the readers of this book will still be around in 30 years and I hope that you will work toward keeping the growth of the cost of health care down without limiting advances in medicine that can save lives and prolong the quality of life as well. If we don't contain the increases in the cost of health care there will be little left for other worthy activities such as education (Fuchs, 2008, p. 1749). Hopefully, because it is an ethical and moral obligation, all people in the United States will be covered, whether it is through the complex Patient Protection and Affordable Care Act, with all its moving parts, or a simple system of single payer and universal coverage, as we find in Canada, with providers essentially not part of the government, subject to some regulations as a utility would be in the United States, and few out-of-pocket costs to limit access to needed services.

The cost issue remains salient in public opinion surveys, even when there are substantially large numbers of people who buy the audacious lies that this is a government-run health care program, much like the Soviet Union in 1950. Clearly, according to tracking polls conducted prior to the 2008 presidential election, concern about the cost of health care became a major issue for voters, with almost half (47%) of those surveyed reporting do at least one of the following:

• Postponed getting care (36%)
• Skipped a recommended medical test or treatment (31%)
• Didn't fill a prescription (27%)
• Cut pills or skipped doses of medicine (22%)
• Had problems getting mental health care (12%)

This national survey did not control for whether respondents had chronic conditions but the budgetary strains of the Great Recession were felt in October 2008 and the cry for help was heard throughout the land. With one in five having medical bills of $1,000 or more, and with few Americans have an adequate savings to take care of unexpected bills, there was a need for health care reform to lower costs to consumers (Kaiser Family Foundation, 2009). Who to help first became an issue during the formulation of two similar bills in the House and the Senate because family finances were hurting to the point that needed care was put on hold. In states where Child Health Plus was available, parents often tried to limit their monthly premiums by only registering the child who had a serious chronic disease or needed corrective surgery while hoping that other children with insurance remained among the well part of the population.

The State Child Health Insurance Program became law during the second Clinton administration because employers were not offering family-based health insurance or at unaffordable prices. Still, a good but declining percentage of health care for working people with chronic illness or family members who are beneficiaries of employer-sponsored insurance are covered by the third-party payer. Premiums are usually shared between the employer and the employee, with an increasing share of the premium being borne by the employee as health care costs continue to rise. For much of the population, a chronic condition means more trips to the doctor and consequently more expenses. With private insurance coverage, the proportion of the bill paid for an outpatient visit by insurance is usually less than what is paid for a hospital stay. In addition, doctor's charges while in the hospital are more likely to see a higher percentage paid by the health plan than going toward the deductable or copayments.

## DECREASING COVERAGE AND ACA REMEDIES

The facts are that working people and their dependents currently are finding substantial barriers to health care produced by the way it is financed; it has become unaffordable to people of modest means. While health care costs continue to rise, there is no comparable increase in income for working people to pay for it. For the past two decades, disparities between those at the top and those at the bottom of income distribution continue to widen, but I digress. There is significant new information on health care insurance coverage and cost disparities that deserves attention by policymakers.

The New York State Health Foundation (NYSHF) reported on November 17, 2010, that a study it commissioned about New York State employer-sponsored health insurance that covers a large part of the working population and their families, as well as early retirees, found that coverage has been declining during the last decade. Since 2001, the percentage of eligible employees in private firms in the Empire State covered by health insurance declined from 85 to 74 percent in 2009. And the take-up of insurance by workers has dropped from 82 to 78 percent (Gabel, Whitmore, and Pickreign, 2010). As a result, the percentage of New York workers with employer-sponsored insurance fell from 69 percent in 2003 to 58 percent in 2009.

If we just focus on the downward trending take-up rate for employer-based insurance, it is not hard to account for why this is happening. According to the NYSHF study, employee contributions through premiums, deductibles, and copays for family coverage doubled from 2001 to 2009 to an average of $3,753. This burden makes people with insurance worry. Nationally, the Robert Wood Johnson Foundation follows a randomly selected national panel of consumers as well as new respondents to the survey and the results for October 2010 showed a decline in confidence in the area of health care because of cost concerns from the September findings (Robert Wood Johnson Foundation, 2010).

But wait, there's more! There is confirmation from a Commonwealth Fund survey of consumers in 11 countries, conducted in the spring and released on November 18, 2010 (Schoen, Osborn, Squires, Doty, Person, and Applebaum, 2010), that one out of three adults in the United States sample goes without medical care because of costs, spent more than $1,000 annually in out-of-pocket cost and had problems with insurance companies and had to spend many hours seeking to determine payer responsibilities. Additionally, one in five Americans had serious financial problems due to health-related problems and were unable to pay their health care bills. These survey reports on problems related to access to care and costs experienced by Americans, in comparison with the other 10 countries sampled, were substantially greater. These are some of the implications of underinsurance as well as uninsurance.

There are remedies available and help is on the way. True, not all these problems will go away when the many parts of the ACA are implemented, but the Act does have far-reaching benefits, including federal assistance for an expansion of Medicaid eligibility in every state, access to the state-based insurance exchanges so that small businesses can locate plans that offer affordable coverage. State-based insurance exchanges also pool individuals, some of whom will be self-employed, so they can purchase affordable individual policies at group prices.

Moving forward, ACA will attempt to lower the growth of the cost of health care by promoting greater access to primary care. And more integrated health care systems, also in the planning stage now, will yield better value for the health-care dollar, mostly by reducing mistakes such as hospital-acquired infections and unnecessary readmissions to recently discharged patients.

The ACA met a rough patch in the road to mandatory insurance as a result of conservative judges rejecting the right of Congress to extend its regulation to interstate commerce where supposedly no action is being taken by those who refuse to buy insurance coverage. The libertarian argument is that the federal government has no right to tell citizens what to buy and health insurance is often a purchase. This narrow interpretation may get these cases to the United States Supreme Court prior to 2014 when the regulations of the Affordable Care Act requires that most Americans carry some kind of health insurance.

I argue strongly in these pages for mandatory coverage because of the complexity of a decision to forgo this purchase in an age when many aspects of living are related, even if they may not appear to be to strictly literate interpreters of the Constitution. There are many unexpected turns to life that need to be addressed proactively. If we can guarantee in advance that we will not get sick or injured and wind up using health care facilities that are paid for by people who buy insurance or have received public insurance from Medicaid or Medicare, then I would say that HCA goes too far. But we cannot guarantee that we won't take a free ride on the coverage provided by someone else that helps keep these facilities open. The failure to purchase insurance is a decision that affects the rates charged by insurance companies across state lines and therefore should be regulated. The alternative is for those who refuse to buy insurance to put up a bond that would be tapped into when needed. How much to put up probably could be established by actuaries but how many who refuse to buy insurance can come up with the amount required? They would need to receive a subsidy, which they would be entitled to under the terms and conditions of the ACA. If refuseniks wind up paying the fine or tax for not purchasing insurance, they will be getting a bargain. Meanwhile, the financing of health care today deserves attention because of the burdens it places on people who need chronic care.

## PERSONAL FINANCING OF CHRONIC CARE

Increasing, people with chronic illnesses are feeling the financial stress of out-of-pocket costs, often a result of shifting of responsibility by employers to employees so they can keep the premiums down for group policies. Using data from the 2007 (17,800 interviews) and 2003 (46,600 interviews) Health Tracking Household Survey, a study conducted by the Center for Studying Health System Change and funded by the Robert Wood Johnson Foundation, Peter Cunningham (2010) noted that there was "a high probability of having medical bill problems is also associated with having poor health and chronic conditions" (p. 11). The economic downturn meant that financial pressures for these families increased over time. With consumer indebtedness rising from 110 percent of personal income to 130 percent in 2007 and foreclosures increasing a stunning 150 percent from 2005 to 2007, there is little surprise that respondents in poor health who participated in this telephone survey experienced hard times. For many of the respondents in this national survey, their coverage was limited. In 2014, to some extent, low and modest income families that purchase health care insurance policies from the state exchanges will get some relief from burdensome medical bills through provisions in the Affordable Care Act that will limit their out-of-pocket expenses according to their incomes.

The issue of being underinsured has been examined more closely with regard to children with serious chronic illnesses and disabilities because of the interest shown in this subject by the Maternal and Child Health Bureau in its advocacy efforts for children and its willingness to fund researchers with considerable experience with doing secondary analyses of data sets of national samples. The concern among policy experts on child health is that this population needs to be monitored closely to make sure they get appropriate care. Ambulatory care is particularly important for children. Onerous out-of-pocket payments and limited access to benefits due to coverage restraints has produced a condition that has been characterized as underinsurance.

This condition has been particularly evident in reports collected in the most recent national survey of children's health, which included questions for parents related to costs of care, benefits related to the child's needs, and whether access to sources of care the child needs was supported by the family's insurance coverage. Therefore, even when insurance was in place, the inadequacy of the coverage could compromise whether a child had access to a medical home. According to authors of an analysis of the 2007 National Survey of Children's Health data, based on a sample of 91,642, almost 23 percent of children with continuous insurance were underinsured because care was deemed inadequate and did not meet the criteria of a medical home because of the following responses to the survey:

- Delayed or forgone care
- Difficult obtaining needed care from a specialist
- No preventive care
- No developmental screening at a preventive visit
- Doctors not spending enough time with the child
- Doctors not listening carefully to the parent
- Doctors insensitive to the family's values and customs
- Doctors not furnishing needed information
- Doctors not making the parent feel like a partner

According to the authors' estimations, there are 14.1 million children with continuous insurance coverage who were underinsured, disproportionately including children in fair or poor health and with special health care needs as well as children from minority groups (Kogan et al., 2010). Note that this number does not include an additional 11 million children who were identified in the survey as not being covered by any insurance. By 2009, at the height of the economic downturn, 50.7 million Americans of all ages were identified as uninsured. At the same time, the number of Americans covered by private insurance, whether through employment, associations that offered group policies for purchase, or through individually purchased policies, declined.

Health care nationally has become a growing financial burden to all Americans, not just the poor as employers shift more and more of the premium costs of policies to employees. Recent reports suggest that the costs are placing a heavy load on families: "almost 30 percent of the U.S. population either had a high financial burden of health costs or were uninsured" (Cunningham, 2010, p. 1038). Trends of this kind, based on data collected for the period 2001 to 2006, mean that incomes do not keep pace with health-care expenditures and there is less in the household budget to take care of other needs. What might the data look like for the period 2007 to 2012, a time when incomes were down and unemployment was up substantially?

The people in the United States with chronic conditions, whether covered by insurance or uninsured, are vulnerable to high out-of-pocket costs that endanger their financial stability and well-being. Peter J. Cunningham (2009) looked closely at the data derived from the 2001–2005 Medical Expenditure Panel Survey for the Commonwealth Fund. When compared with people with single chronic conditions and those with no chronic conditions, 40 percent of people with three or more chronic conditions had out-of-pocket expenses and premiums exceeding 5 percent of income. Among those with single chronic conditions, 20 percent had costs beyond 5 percent of income while 14 percent of those who reported no chronic conditions had health care expenditures that came to 5 percent of their income.

There were persistently high expenses for 39 percent of those with multiple chronic illnesses for two consecutive years (Cunningham, 2009, p. 3). I know from my own experience as a 71-year-old person with a chronic illness, hypertension, from being followed quarterly after prostate cancer surgery, additional quarterly visits to detect any new skin cancers, as well as annually visits to the ophthalmologist to monitor my corneal dystrophy, there are some expensive laboratory tests and high-tech in-office diagnostic procedures that are my responsibility financially because of the large deductible in my employer-issued health insurance coverage as well as copays for office visits.

These personal out-of-pocket expenses are paralleled by the high price of Lipitor, the only brand name medication that I take, although there are now generics available and I switched to one of them in 2011. So in my case, as well as a good part of the population above the age of 55, some of these continuous costs related to the use of prescription drugs, identified as the single largest contributor to financial burdens for individuals, account for 55 percent of the costs for those with two or more conditions. In addition, because individually written policies are less generous than group policies usually issued at the workplace, when chronic illness occurs, those with individual coverage are likely to have the greatest out-of-pocket expenditures. In some states, such as California, there are extreme exclusions of people with preexisting conditions and, consequently, the premiums are low. However, low premiums also means that what is covered in the way of benefits is also quite limited (Rau, 2008). Additionally, as shown with Anthem of California during the run-up to the signing of the Affordable Care Act, the premiums have become unaffordable for many young people who are well but out of work or underpaid and they have dropped coverage, leading to a request by this insurer in 2010 for a rate increase close to 40 percent.

Premiums are also kept low when there is cost sharing. Copays are designed to keep the "worried well" out of the doctor's office and thereby reduce health care utilization. However, there are unintended health consequences when individuals who should be seen by a doctor and perhaps receive some additional services (e.g., nutritional guidance) are forced to make a decision about having to see the doctor and pay perhaps $25 for the visit or limiting the number of visits made for primary or specialty care. Many of us get angry at ourselves when we make an office visit and the physician says what you think you have is nothing to worry about. People of modest means with chronic illnesses may avoid visits to doctors and therefore avoid copays, resulting in shifting the cost of care from ambulatory services to hospital care.

People with one or more chronic illness may be particularly vulnerable to the efforts to reduce or shift the cost of health care to the consumer. The trend for employers is to make available only high-deductible health plans based on preferred provider organizations, where participating hospitals and physicians contract to give significant discounts to the insurer. These discounts are passed on to employers who purchase coverage but also limit the premiums they pay by requiring participating employees to assume a high deductible before indemnification is triggered. In the largest statewide health survey conducted in California, the UCLA Center for Health Policy Research found that between the years 2003 to 2007, affordability counts. State residents in plans with high deductibles often went without care because of the out-of-pocket payments they were required to make as part of their managed care plan (Simmons, 2010). In addition, "Low-income residents were more likely to have health plans with excessive out-of-pocket costs—as were 32% of low-income earners enrolled in PPOs, the report found. And some 38% of those individually insured, with no employer-based healthcare coverage, were also members of high deductible healthcare plans" (Simmons, 2010).

There are some kinds of coverage that promote community care. Medicare Advantage plans offer a wide variety of benefits but often have copays. Even among 899,000 people who are in these managed care plans and who were followed for five years, between 2001 and 2006, and where an increase in copayments for ambulatory care took place, in the year following the increases in cost sharing for both for primary and specialty care, there was a sharp reduction in the use of ambulatory services. Limiting visits to the doctor, the goal of copays, does not always benefit patients who may wind up being hospitalized when their medical condition deteriorates. The results are quite striking: Plans that increased cost sharing had 19.8 fewer annual outpatient visits per 100 enrollees, an additional 2.2 hospital admissions, and 13.4 more annual inpatient days per 100 enrollees. As the authors of this study convincingly point out, "The effects of increases in copayments for ambulatory care were magnified among enrollees living in areas of lower income and education and among enrollees who had hypertension, diabetes, or a history of myocardial infarction" (Trivedi, Moloo, and Mor, 2010, p. 210).

Therefore, there is a warning to be issued concerning this attempt to lower premiums. The user of health benefits beware. A New York State based study of cost sharing concluded that "The increase in cost sharing decreases the financial protection that insurance provides an individual with serious or chronic illnesses, blurring the distinction between group and individual coverage, since individuals covered in the group retain more of their individual risk through out-of-pocket costs" (United Hospital Fund, 2010, p. 19).

The myriad ways of creating insurance coverage in the United States is a nightmare from the point of view of providers who must file claims to get paid for services rendered. Prior authorizations for access to specialists also create an administrative headache since forms must be filled out for the patient by the doctor or the doctor's support staff. It is reported widely by insurance companies and medical executives that administration accounts for 30 percent of all health care expenditures in the United States. The nurses and other professionals who work in medical practices claim that their administrative workload has doubled in the past five years. Just getting the insurance companies to pay in a timely manner also means that payrolls are hard to meet in group practices or hospitals (Costello, Girion, and Hiltzik, 2008).

Providers are not the only ones with financing issues. The availability of expensive drugs is a result of advances in medicine that are praiseworthy. However, not every expensive prescription has been shown to be effective in treating either individuals with a single or those with several comorbidities. There needs to be more emphasis in finding out what works and under what conditions, as we saw earlier in reviewing the likelihood that chemotherapy will work on all tumors that generate certain types of cancers. Funds for studying the effectiveness of treatments and medical practices were part of ARRA, the 2009 stimulus package passed by Congress and signed into law by the president in the spring of that year. We should be seeing results shortly from this investment.

Those with chronic illnesses under the age of 65 are often medically indigent, a term used to describe people with limited income and resources and big medical bills. They sometimes can become Medicaid eligible, depending on how low the bar is set in each state. If individuals qualify for the income maintenance program, Supplemental Security Disability Income, as mentioned earlier, because they cannot work and are declared disabled, then they can be eligible for Medicare prior to the age of 65.

Some individuals will fall between the cracks and will not be eligible for full access to any public health insurance programs. There is going to be a substantial part of this pre-Medicare low- and moderate-income population that does not have either private or public insurance and will still not qualify for Medicaid. They will require subsidization to get their medical bills paid. To help keep the cost of insurance low, if we turn to commercial insurance to issue policies for a population that has preexisting conditions, they will have to be offset by insurance coverage for healthy people below the age of 65 who will pay some of the premium for individual coverage but will be profitable for the insurance companies to issue policies. Without mandatory but partially subsidized coverage, this healthy and younger part of the population will seek to avoid the monthly payments for health insurance. Some with low incomes will be eligible for subsidies based on income and others will access public insurance in all states, including those that previously excluded single adults from Medicaid. Some states have threatened to leave the Medicaid program entirely if they are required to insure this part of the low-income population, even though this would mean losing what they are already collecting from the federal treasury as well as new payments.

The Affordable Care Act will increase eligibility for Medicaid in 2014, making it possible for 16 million low-income adults and children to receive coverage. Providing both affordable and comprehensive coverage for many people with chronic illnesses and disabilities, Medicaid will now insure those with incomes below 133 percent of the poverty line, or approximately $14,000 for an individual. The assets possessed by an individual will not be considered in determining eligibility, making it possible for people with small bank accounts or insurance policies to hold on to them when they become Medicaid beneficiaries. During the first three years in which these changes to

Medicaid are in effect, the federal government will pay 100 percent of the costs for medical and health services for these new eligibles, with a phase down that will mean that by 2020, the states will pick up 10 percent of the financing (Solomon, 2010). Under this plan there will be limited copays and deductibles, unlike most commercial insurance plans.

How well do highly regarded health plans, such as the Federal Employees Health Benefits Plan's Blue Cross and Blue Shield standard option, protect the beneficiary from major out-of-pocket expenses when serious chronic illnesses such as stage III colon cancer, the third most common type of cancer found among both men and women, need to be treated? The American Cancer Society Cancer Action Network commissioned the Georgetown University Health Policy Institute to determine if this policy produced adequate insurance in the case of a serious chronic condition. The plan capped total patient cost-sharing expenses at $5,000 a year if the preferred provider network was utilized for care and $7,000 annually if the patient went outside the network. The analysis found that for all the conditions and there treatments reviewed, the plan had an actuarial value of 90 percent, roughly similar to other employer-sponsored group plans. This means that it appears that the plan is designed mainly to afford protection against major medical expenses if a covered person requires massive interventions over a long period of time (Georgetown University Health Policy Institute, 2009).

For the less than healthy, especially those with several chronic conditions, whether among the elderly or the nonelderly, but highlighted by growth in multiple chronic illnesses among people in midlife, out-of-pocket spending continues to go up. During the last 10 years, not only has the prevalence of chronic illness increased, according to the 2005 Medical Expenditure Panel Survey, but there has been an overall increase of out-of-pocket spending by 39.4 percent on average per person. This astounding increase masks the fact that for some in the survey, out-of-pocket expenditures can be double or triple the average. As I am prone to say, there is no such thing as an average person since averages are constructs from large numbers of people. Certainly lifestyle changes could reduce this increase in the presence of chronic conditions but expansion of access to care for nonelderly adults most certainly is required, given the needs identified in the survey (Paez, Zhao, and Hwang, 2009, pp. 15–25).

Making this right will be driven by health care reform legislation passed in 2010. Some Americans today are refused coverage because of their chronic conditions. The stories told by these individuals helped sell the Affordable Care Act to the U.S. public and there was no lack of stories to tell. The magnitude of the problem is widespread and what makes the ACA a source of potent reforms in many states. The diagnoses of some 57 million, or one in five people under the age of 65, according to the progressive advocacy group Family USA, are screened out of the insurance market by states that do not require guaranteed issue in the individual insurance policy market. There is also evidence collected by state insurance commissions that have had policies canceled because beneficiaries were experiencing serious and expensive bouts of illness and were therefore expensive to the company that issued the policy. In September 2010, the ACA eliminated the practice of rescinding policies. There is also hope that by 2014, the new law of the land will prevent the denial of issuing policies because of preexisting conditions. The average annual cost of policies will increase some 14 percent but benefits will also improve substantially.

In addition, all policies will provide an array of benefits that make the coverage package a worthwhile purchase. From the point of view of a person with a serious chronic illness, at least chronic disease management, if not a patient-centered medical home, will be covered, along with doctor visits, hospital care, mental health and substance abuse services, benefits currently found in good employer-based packages. Employer-based insurance plans, to save money, have become more and more limited when it comes to these necessary services and thereby irrelevant as a source of security.

In addition, choice of plan according to payment responsibilities under the state insurance exchanges will also help people with chronic care needs. Those who anticipate heavy use of services can select a plan that will pay higher premiums but will receive in the "platinum plan," coverage for 90 percent of their costs. All policies issued under the ACA will have no lifetime or annual caps on expenditures, something that people with chronic illnesses can appreciate. Moreover, reform in the individual insurance market will cap out-of-pocket costs at $5,950 for an individual and $11,900 for a family annually. To promote equity, lower-income families will meet their annual out-of-pocket costs in the form of deductibles and copayments at a lower total dollar amount (Rabin, 2010b, p. 6).

In the years leading up to 2014, to create some security, individuals who were previously denied coverage because of preexisting conditions will be able to buy into preexisting condition plans. These plans are considered bridges to the time when exclusions will not be permitted. The federal government is supplying payments to states that have what are known as high-risk plans or are establishing such plans in states that did not have them but also prevented insurers from excluding individuals from purchasing commercial insurance on the open market. Usually, there will be a waiting period of six months for eligible individuals who had no credible coverage to become eligible as well as prove via documentation that they have preexisting condition before they can buy insurance. In some states, such as Illinois and New York, the Department of Health and Human Services will contract directly with an exclusive provider program (Hayes, 2010).

So the problem of how to provide medical care for the chronically ill is clearly tied to the more generic problem of how to have quality care for everyone at a reasonable cost. Victor Fuchs (2008), a long-time advocate of the social insurance model of health care coverage, suggests that progressive taxation, or basically income transfer, is important in making sure that everyone has access to care regardless of capacity to pay or the cost of care.

> The most efficient, equitable way to achieve universal coverage is to make basic health insurance available to everyone regardless of income, employment status, family circumstances, or other characteristics and to pay for it with a tax roughly proportional to income or consumption. In such a system, the wealthy and the healthy would subsidize insurance for the poor and the sick. Persons of average income and average health would pay enough to cover the cost of their own insurance. (p. 1751)

## FINDING THE BEST BUY

Yet, despite the simplicity and fairness of such a plan, it does not mention that the cost of care continues to rise, driven largely by expensive technological innovations or new drug therapies, many of which do not make much of a difference compared to what are already standard treatment options. Payers such as Medicare will cover charges for treatments no matter what the costs as long as they are regarded as effective, even when there are equally effective and less-costly options already in place. David Leonhardt (2010b), a business columnist, describes the three options for treating prostate cancer with radiation, all producing good outcomes but at enormous variation in price. He endorses a plan devised by two doctors, both former Medicare officials, Steven Pearson and Peter B. Bach, and both currently affiliated with nationally recognized cancer centers at Massachusetts General Hospital and Memorial Sloan Kettering Cancer Center, respectively, that would "give expensive new treatments three years to prove that they work better than cheaper treatments, or their reimbursement rates would be cut to that of the cheaper treatments" (p. B1).

Facing the kind of restriction proposed by Pearson and Bach would be similar mind concentrating functions as contemplating the gallows. I anticipate that treatment centers that consider utilizing radiological treatment innovations might hesitate before making the investment to install big ticket items that might not generate the revenues that would make them profit centers. Having to prove that an expensive treatment is a race to the top in terms of better results could put a damper to what amounts to a nuclear arms race that is going on in cancer treatment.

Some payers are moving swiftly to rein in costs in cancer care and are not waiting for the results of studies supported by the Center for Patient Centered Effectiveness Research to see the light of day. Some commercial insurers such as UnitedHealthCare are creating financial incentives for oncologists to choose the least-expensive chemotherapy available, rather than selecting the expensive customized or even unproven therapeutic alternatives. Peter B. Bach notes that Medicare will pay for eight different chemotherapy treatments for lung cancer that vary in cost per month from $7,092 (Pernetrexed) to $1,322 (Paclitaxel) (Abelson, 2010b, p. B8).

Similarly, pharmaceutical manufacturers might also have second thoughts before scaling up production of a blockbuster drug that does not show decisive advantages of the less expensive but equally good drug already widely prescribed. Less risky innovations are efforts to bring on line the financing of advanced primary care.

## STRUCTURING PAYMENTS FOR MEDICAL HOMES AND BRINGING THEM TO SCALE

Some of the more adventurous efforts in patient-centered care, as presented earlier with regard to accountable care organizations such as the Mount Auburn, Massachusetts, partnership, also depend on new ways of financing that allow for the creation of performance incentives that support ambulatory care without punishing the hospital. An alternative quality contract with Blue Cross and Blue Shield of Massachusetts permitted hospitals to get rewarded for not admitting patients when they showed up at the emergency department (ED) but reconnecting them to their primary care practitioners (PCP). When tests were run, whether during a hospital stay or an ED visit, they were reported to the PCP, helping to avoid future unnecessary hospital admissions (Commonwealth Fund, 2010, p. 7).

Sometimes the focus of changing how primary care providers deliver chronic care focuses on one highly prevalent disease, such as diabetes in Germany, where a disease management program was launched to address the problem. The German insurance system was struck by the fact that about 14.2 percent of total spending in the health care system was on patients with diabetes. The single largest sickness fund in Germany created a countrywide disease management program for diabetes, with 19,882 enrollees (Stock et al., 2010, p. 2198). So convinced were the policymakers in Germany that something had to be done to reduce expenditures, this new program was initiated nationally without the benefit of small pilot programs to establish its viability.

The program works through participating "physicians [who] coordinate care across disciplines and professions in accordance with an individualized treatment plan based on evidence-based care goals" (Stock et al., 2010, p. 2198). The patient's health profile and attendant risks are the basis for determining the lump-sum payment. All sickness funds pay into a "Risk Compensation Scheme" so that funds that have a disproportionately high percentage of the insured with chronic diseases will receive additional payments to offset their additional indemnifications for services delivered by these primary care physicians (Stock et al., 2010, p. 2198).

On the other side of the equation, patients are incentivized by the elimination of copayments for these disease management services when they sign up with a primary-care provider. The participating patients must attend diabetes education classes and agree to show up for regular follow-up visits with these doctors. Comparative effectiveness research was carried out for this large population. When these patients, all volunteers, were compared with patients with similar age, gender, and health characteristics, the research team found that the overall mortality rate and the occurrence of significant secondary conditions such as myocardial infarction, stroke, chronic renal insufficiency, and infections of the lower leg and foot were lower for the intervention group than the control group. The main cost difference between the intervention and the control group was related to the fact that those patients receiving this innovative primary care service were less likely to be hospitalized and when admitted to the hospital, stayed for fewer days than those who received the routine care available. Patients in the intervention group had better control over their diabetes and hypertension, resulting in fewer deaths during the study period (Stock et al., 2010, p. 2201).

And there is strong evidence that the patient-centered medical home approach, as adapted by German health insurance system, is needed in other countries with universal coverage. We have reports from Canada, the country with a single payer system that guarantees universal coverage and access to primary care for the entire population, that the delivery system, at least in one province, Ontario, benefited from some redesign work that created patient-centered medical homes. Following the lead of the United States, the province health care authorities realized that the payment system was encouraging high-volume practices, despite the higher ratio of primary care to specialty care in Canada. As of 2010, using a blended payment model and delivering services via 150 Family Health Teams (FHT), a million patients are served through 750 physicians.

To get family physicians in Ontario to partner in Family Health Teams, the province boosted the income for family physicians from $180,000 to $250,000 (Canadian) while the family physicians in fee-for-service practice saw no increase in income. According to Rosser and his associates' e-article (2010), the payment for participating family physicians is based on age- and sex-based capitation. For example, a doctor who had a large number of people over 75 years of age would get extra payments. Bonuses were also made available for physicians who set prevention goals for a panel of patients. One comparative study found that hypertension rates were better controlled through the Family Health Teams than through routine but unmanaged fee-for-service visits.

Higher pay and the family approach was a recruiting tool and helped to address shortages in primary care. The FHT program has had a positive impact on Ontario's medical school graduates entering the field of primary care, with an increase from 25 percent in 2004 to 79 percent in 2009. In contrast, other provinces did not show such spectacular gains. Yet Ontario reported that even family physicians in practice for many years are starting to convert to the FHT model.

In a lesser studied innovation by virtue of its location in a rapidly developing country—Brazil—the government is not only extending coverage to all its citizens but is engaged in a major expansion of primary care through packaging that is similar to patient-centered medical homes. The financial foundation for this effort is through government support of community health clinics, where the Family Health Program teams are based and through which they deliver services. Home visits and health promotion activities are carried out by a team that consists of one physician, one nurse, one medical assistant, and four to six community health agents. These teams have an enormous reach, by 2007 furnishing community health services to 99.4 million people, a bit greater than half of the country's population. Starting in 1999 with 4,114 units, the Family Health Program grew so rapidly that by 2007 there were more than 29,000 in the field. Consequently, with this kind of scale, The Family Health Program constitutes the largest community-based primary care service on the planet (Macinko et al., 2010, pp. 2149–2150). There is a bit of history that accounts for this growth in services.

Since the 1960s, Brazil has experienced a large increase in the prevalence of chronic diseases, so that by 2005, the leading cause of death, accounting for 30 percent of all deaths, was cardiovascular disease. Cancer accounted for 15 percent of all death that year and diabetes-related deaths doubled since 1990. Brazil responded by forming the Family Health Program and targeted cardiovascular disease and diabetes prevention and treatment, using clinical practice guidelines and community health education programs to introduce changes in lifestyle that can prevent the onset of these diseases or mitigate increasing severity (Macinko et al., 2010, p. 2150).

Researchers in Brazil followed the impact of the Family Health Program by measuring both death rates nationally and the extent to which there was a reduction of ambulatory care sensitive hospitalizations related to chronic illnesses by age group and sex. Since 1999, the rates of hospitalization of hypertension, stroke, other cardiovascular diseases, and chronic obstructive pulmonary disease dropped significantly. Moreover, there was evidence that the resulting reduction in the utilization of scarce and expensive health care resources was due to the availability of the community-based teams sent out through the Family Health Program. Where the percentage of enrollments in municipalities in the Family Health Program was high, there were lower rates of hospital admissions and lower lengths of stay than in those municipalities where fewer citizens received their care from these community-based units (Macinko et al., 2010, p. 2154).

There were some limits to this study. First, not all results in the study pointed in the same direction. In a surprise finding, the rate of hospitalization of diabetes increased through access to the Family Health Program teams, perhaps because they found people with diabetes in these municipalities who had neglected diabetes care and required hospital admission to receive interventions with difficult conditions. Second, the researchers also acknowledged that beyond comparing rates of hospitalization over time and better localities that had varying access to the teams, they did not seek to develop indicators of the quality of the primary care delivered and its impact (Macinko et al., 2010, p. 2156).

What is happening in Germany, Canada, and Brazil is what is called capacity building or scaling up, a sustained transformation of primary care so it receives more financing and becomes more attractive to future doctors. Hopefully, these doctors and U.S. medical school graduates will not only have a new concept of what it means to be a physician in the twenty-first century but also will receive the compensation that is justifiable, given the effort that they will put in building up the PCMH. Getting to that point requires a profound understanding that primary care involves more than patient visits, using a vision of service that goes beyond that encounter but also is built around a sense of responsibility for maintaining the relationship with the patient. Much of this planning and execution involves creating a financial platform for the PCMH that also is aligned with tertiary care at the medical center. Horner and Baron (2010) argue eloquently that moving forward this is the only kind of care that is appropriate in our time.

> For transformation of primary care to become widespread, the transformation cannot be limited to primary care offices but must also include payment reform, widespread application of health information technology, creation of shared community resources, engagement of a broader set of health professionals (especially nursing) and major changes in the roles and relationships between primary care and the other components of the health care system. (p. 626)

The patient-centered medical home requires both start-up and maintenance funding to make available electronic medical records for all patients as well as targeted funding to take into account that patient fees will not compensate fairly for the additional time required for some patients. Care management for colocated chronic conditions, with the additional consults with specialists, additional nurses, and social workers, and the time required to teach self-management skills to people with serious chronic illnesses are expenses required for patient-centered medical homes to make a difference in the lives of patients (Merrell and Berenson, 2010, p. 853). With more experience with caring for the chronically ill in patient-centered medical homes, a result of capacity building, it will be easier to determine how to align costs.

The hope of financing experts is that there is a foundation of information available to make appropriate payments for chronic care in the patient-centered medical home possible.

> [B]ecause common risk-adjustment approaches rely on diagnosis information generally obtained from submitted claims, it is logical, although not yet demonstrated, that risk adjusted comprehensive payments could be applied at the medical home level. (Merrell and Berenson, 2010, p. 856)

The financial plight of underinsured people with chronic illnesses will not go away without some tinkering with the insurance and payment system of this country. Nevertheless, this is an exciting time for validating the importance of the medical home and the recovery of primary care from its secondary position in health care in America. There are some roadblocks to these changes, however, which appear when we look at both undergraduate and graduate medical education, as well as for the greater deployment of advanced practice nurses. In the next chapter, I will examine the shortfall in primary care in the United States, largely because it dwells in the shadow of specialty care, both in terms of prestige and income.

# 8

# The Primary Care and Medical Home Shortfall: A Wakeup Call for an Aging Society

When I wrote the first draft of this chapter, President Obama had posted on February 22, 2010, his health care reform proposal on the official whitehouse.gov website in an effort to unify his party and get the Senate and the House to support a proposal that is a hybrid of both their bills. While the focus of the proposal is permitting U.S. families and small businesses to control their own health care by establishing subsidies for the low-income uninsured in the United States, there has to be support to build capacity to deliver services to the estimated 37 million newly insured who in the past had limited access to medical care.

Driven largely by the progressive wing of the Democratic Party, the House bill contained a specific item that supported increased access to preventive and primary health services and was an allocation of $12.5 billion for new community health centers. The Senate bill, in contrast, allocated $7 billion for community health centers. These centers are not new to the United States. Community health centers were started in 1962 to assist migrant workers in rural communities. During the Bush 43 Administration, to its credit, the funding was doubled from what was appropriated during the Clinton Administration and there are now 1,250 centers that serve 20 million people, many of whom are uninsured or Medicaid recipients. There is also additional funding for community health centers to reorganize and upgrade their services so they can then be deemed Federally Qualified by the Department of Health and Human Services.

To support more health centers and to increase the numbers of primary care providers in underserved areas of the country, the proposal supports through the National Health Service Corps substantial funding of scholarships and loan repayment for doctors, nurses, and other health professionals who will then practice in rural and urban areas designated as underserved because of provider shortages. In addition, scholarships and loan repayments will be available for eligible disadvantaged students who commit to working in areas where there are shortages of medical services.

In addition, on June 16, 2010, Secretary Sebelius announced that federal funding in the amount of $250 million to help provide training to more than 16,000 primary care providers in the next five years. The Medicare payment gap between specialists and primary care providers would also be reduced through a 10 percent bonus for the same period.

Given these incentives, will the medical schools take into account the need for increased education and training in primary care and geriatric medicine so that there will be a supply of doctors who can work with patients with multiple chronic illnesses? Will physicians be sufficiently comfortable in the chronic care encounter, when a patient is in need of being located in a patient-centered medical home, or is facing physical decline, to be able to undertake the analytic and interpersonal processes necessary to help the individual?

Currently, it is hard to imagine that such a contact will take place. In the three-year period from 2007 to 2009, fewer than 100 U.S. medical school graduates opted for postdoctoral training in geriatrics (Cassel, 2009, p. 2701). In an aging society, with the well-known Baby Boom generation reaching the ripe old age when Social Security pensions are issued, this is hardly a sufficient number of doctors to deal with the emerging need. A study conducted by the Institute of Medicine, a federal agency, reported in 2008 that there is an acute shortage of geriatricians now and going forward (Committee on the Future Health Care Workforce for Older Americans, 2008). There does not seem to be a plan in place to overcome this shortage.

Where are students going to learn geriatrics in an interdisciplinary setting? The options are few and far between. Gaining the knowledge, ability, and motivation to deliver these services is a down payment on the future. Geriatric clinics would be the likely loci for the development of this area of expertise. Too often, these programs are closed when continued support is withdrawn from state and municipal sources. Programs of this kind cannot be put in the "shovel ready" category—they cannot be started up and perform at full capacity in a short period of time. These programs are repositories of human and social capital that are needed to promote the use of evidence-based services if we are to adequately train the next generation of primary care providers.

Capacity building, as with any institutional development, is required for meeting immediate and future needs. There is no substitute for well-trained primary care providers who are capable of delivering proven-to-be effective services and increasing the efficacy of new interventions. While primary care does not depend on sophisticated diagnostic or treatment technology, many skilled providers can identify the onset of chronic disease or deterioration and implement evidence-based interventions that can induce savings or cost offsets by reducing the need for subsequent complex and expensive treatments.

Part of the problem for how to address the primary care shortage is a lack of interest among medical students in matching, or doing residencies at hospitals and medical centers in primary care fields, a trend that continues to show drops in applications from medical school graduates, from 55.8 percent in 1998 to 40 percent in 2009. The shrinkage in the number of health maintenance organizations that rely heavily on primary care providers means fewer future opportunities available. Yet there is also a medical culture to contend with, according to one medical student with a frustrating experience in attempting to maintain diet compliance for a diabetic patient. Ishani Ganguli (2010) maintains that

> there is an overwhelming ethos of subspecialization at academic medical centers like Harvard. The predominance of specialists among our teachers reflects a health care system that affords such practitioners more money and prestige, and we students are subtly and frequently entreated to get that for ourselves, not to waste our talent. (p. 208)

The distribution of physicians as a labor supply varies from state to state and from locality to locality. There is evidence from a California statewide survey that while physician supply may have grown faster than population since 1998, there are is also a serious shortage of primary-care providers in the Golden State. Six of the nine regions in California do not have the recommended number of primary care physicians. Consequently, the most vulnerable part of the population—people without health insurance and those covered by Medicaid—often have a hard time finding a regular source of care (California Health Care

Foundation Almanac Update, 2010). In addition, in the future, California may face a serious reduction in the number of physicians in practice since this profession has currently in practice a large number of doctors who are older than 60. Perhaps the future increases in Medicare payment rates, made law by the Affordable Care Act, will entice them to stay in practice.

## ADVANCED PRACTICE NURSING AND CHRONIC CARE

Policymakers are starting to note this serious reduction in providers with medical degrees and are taking a different tack to create capacity in primary care, following some federal efforts already in place to expand primary care using nurse practitioners (NPs). Previous legislation, the Medicare Modernization Act and Extension Act of 2006, which originally allowed only physicians to be considered primary care providers, was modified in 2008 to permit NPs to become care coordinators, especially for people with chronic conditions, in the Medical Home Demonstration Expansion. This newly empowered source of primary care, NPs' participation in patient-centered medical homes, was endorsed by the American College of Physicians in 2009 so long as these providers were held to the same eligibility requirements and evaluative standards as medical general practitioners (Schram, 2010). Expansion of the patient-centered medical home will also require more advance practice nurses to do the care coordination for people with chronic illnesses, such as diabetes.

In addition, the primary care shortages that currently exist and are anticipated to be exacerbated by expanding coverage via Medicaid and the state insurance exchanges calls for employing nurse practitioners to deliver safe and effective primary care. Training and education can be quick and inexpensive compared with the daunting regimen for physicians. And more graduates from nurse practitioner programs are required since the annual rate of 8,000 has remained unchanged for several years (Aiken, 2010, p. 1).

Critical to the expansion of the primary care workforce, according to advance practice advocates for the nursing profession, is the elimination of state regulatory restrictions on what nurse practitioners can do. Currently 16 states and the District of Columbia have altered their score-of-practice regulations so that nurse practitioners can prescribe independently (Fairman, Rowe, Hassmiller, and Shalala, 2010, p. 2).

The need for primary care practitioners nationally, and especially to furnish services for Medicaid-eligible individuals, was recognized by the creators of health care reform legislation. The good news is that appropriations through the Affordable Care Act will sustain an enormous leap in the availability of primary care providers. With 5 percent of the current U.S. population receiving health services through a "pay-as-you-can" formula, through community health centers, we are likely to find a way of learning from programs for the poor on how to establish primary care via the patient-centered medical home model. Designed to serve more than migrant workers, the program expanded during the days of the Great Society in 1965 through the Office of Economic Opportunity. With added funding, the community health centers began to zero in on health professional shortage areas, whether in rural or urban areas. One of the founding fathers of one of the first community health centers, Jack Geiger, joins in singing the praises of the potential impact of what will become a major platform for better health care delivery to people with chronic illnesses (Adashi, Geiger, and Fine, 2010, p. 1).

This improvement will be fueled by a major education and training effort nationally. Now with an increase of 15,000 primary care providers expected to be at work by 2016, it is anticipated that 40 million Americans will be getting their care in community health centers (Adashi, Geiger, and Fine, 2010, p. 4). Nevertheless, the policies of those institutions that do graduate medical education, mainly academic medical centers, which serve as teaching hospitals, would have to change if these numeric goals will be meet. Currently, too few primary care physicians are being trained. General support from Medicare for graduate medical education may come under closer review by Congress if the goals set to train more primary care physicians to work in an expanded Medicaid and private insurance are not being met (Iglehart, 2010a, p. 7).

It is not only that the numbers of Americans receiving primary care from this source will double during this decade, but that this affordable care will be comprehensive, coordinated, and patient centered, as well as community accountable and culturally competent. A major hurdle will be access to specialty care when providers often refuse to see patients who are Medicaid eligible or even Medicare eligible because the fees are lower than they expect.

Despite this major challenge, the community health center is built around the idea of the patient-centered medical home, and with it, "a whole person orientation, accessibility, affordability, high quality, and accountability" that could well inform tomorrow's primary care paradigm. And this paradigm is supported by "the use of decision-support tools and ongoing quality measurement and improvement" (Adashi, Geiger, and Fine, 2010, p. 4).

According to Christine Cassel (2009, p. 2701), American health care is a long way away from having the structure and process to produce valuable outcomes with an aging population. Any efforts, she suggests, to reduce the number of hospital readmissions among the Medicare population will require an ambulatory medical workforce that:

- Possesses extensive knowledge of the aging process, prognostic indicators, and the multiple geriatrics syndromes
- Can deliver proactive care that is long term
- Has available a multidisciplinary team as part of the medical practice structure
- Commands good communications skills that can be utilized in personal interaction with the patient, permitting the physicians to take into account his or her values, goals, and preferences
- Establishes continuity across diverse settings so that transitions are benign
- Works with hospitals to reduce risks to elderly patients by increasing awareness of the patient's health status, particularly if fragile, and the dangers of adverse drug interactions

Current cries for expanding the number of students in medical colleges and the number of medical schools in the United States are ways to promote demand for primary care residencies without cutting down on the number of specialty care residencies. To what extent graduate medical education in primary care general practice traineeships such as family medicine, general internal medicine, and general pediatrics will attract graduates with huge medical school debt and the opportunity to earn far less than physicians trained in invasive cardiology, diagnostic radiology, or orthopedic surgery, the specialties with the highest median incomes in the United States, as reported in 2006, does not create a hopeful picture for change. The median salaries for the top three medical specialties, as named above, are close to three times more than the salaries reported by the primary care providers (Iglehart, 2008, p. 648). While the reinvention of primary care is a task too important to fail, Susan Dentzer (2010a), the editor of *Health Affairs*, America's leading journal on health policy, notes that "the net present value of career-long earnings for primary care physicians, at just over $2 million, is about $3 million less than the comparable figure for cardiologists" (p. 757).

The Bush 43 Administration, with its market orientation for the solution of all pressing policy issues, largely stepped out of the debate on how to create more primary care providers, despite significant evidence from other countries that shows that access to primary care generates positive results in terms of healthier patients who live longer. The noninterventionist approach of this administration was not respected by Mark B. McClellan, the administrator for the Centers for Medicare and Medicaid Services from 2004 to 2006, who said,

> There are increasing calls for GME (graduate medical education) reform but that has not translated into broad support for changes that could save some money and provide better support for training physicians in innovative approaches to coordinate care, enhance care for disadvantaged populations and develop better models for translational research. These are vital goals that need further development as soon as possible. (quoted by John K. Iglehart, August 7, 2008, p. 649)

The call for reform in graduate medical education to support primary care has come from a coalition of large employers, consumer groups, and professional associations. Entitled the "patient centered primary care collaborative," this association has kept alive the concept that primary care will become the centerpiece of health care delivery reforms (Iglehart, 2008). As recently as fall 2009, the Patient-Centered Primary Care Collaborative had jump-started 27 multi-stakeholder pilot projects, rolled out in 18 states. Forty four states and the District of Columbia have either passed legislation to enable the primary care medical home practice or have engaged in promoting that kind of activity.

Some caution must be shown when it comes to the efforts to propel primary care forward as the solution to how to supply high-quality care through access alone. Better treatment outcomes, according to a 2010 Dartmouth College study, does not come about simply by getting patients to primary care providers. Based on data from the 2003 to 2007 Medicare records, the researchers found that there was wide variability among patients who were seen by primary care providers as to whether they received standardized recommended diagnostic tests such as mammograms to detect breast cancer and A1c testing to track the management of diabetes through reviewing blood sugar levels (Reichard, 2010c). Regional and state differences in the quality of care were identified in this study.

## STATEWIDE EFFORTS TO INCREASE ACCESS TO PRIMARY CARE

Outside of the area of graduate medical education, the collaborative has also supported systemic (reorganization) changes in health care delivery to improve chronic care. There has been one major attempt to initiate statewide the model of chronic care created by Ed Wagner, the father of the medical home, in the primary care practices of Pennsylvania. With these models in mind, the Governor's Office of Health Care Reform started this three-year initiative in May 2008. Participating stakeholders in the Keystone State include 11 insurance companies as well as several provider-run health systems, professional associations, and government agencies. There are 780 physicians from internal medicine, family medicine, and pediatrics participating. Payments are made to 170 participating practices to help offset practice management costs, the expenses associated with hiring or contracting for care management and incentives to improve clinical quality, demonstrate efficiencies and cost savings, and improve patient satisfaction (Lewis, 2009).

Other states, including Colorado, Michigan, North Carolina, Oklahoma, and Vermont, have introduced initiatives to create networks among solo primary and chronic care providers, to establish agreements between public and private payers, and to establish rewards for positive outcomes in the care of people with chronic illnesses. In addition, states are also supporting team approaches to care, the organization of learning, and information feedback to improve chronic care. Finally, external certifications and recognition through national organizations have been adopted as well as state-driven audits of compliance (Takach, Gauthier, Sims-Kastelein, and Kaye, 2010).

Through the collective efforts of several medical associations, as mentioned earlier, modeling has sought to define the PCMH by its mission, "as a team of people embedded in the community who seek to improve the health and healing of the people in that community." This community orientation is the outcome of PCMH that "personalize, prioritize, and integrate care to improve the health of whole people, families, communities and populations" (Stange et al., 2010, p. 602). Personalized care does count; there is no reason why a specialist, for example, rather than a primary care provider, cannot orchestrate a comprehensive care approach for patients with recondite problems, if that is the best way to go.

This approach seeks to add value to the contact between patient and physician, making it the preferred method for the delivery of health care. Most importantly, when it comes to chronic illness, there is a strong emphasis on the "Integration of care across multiple co-morbid chronic illnesses" (Stange et al., 2010, p. 606). And despite the strong emphasis on gaining value through a redesign of primary care, there is also a need to pay close attention to the consequences, intended and otherwise, of measuring these encounters and introducing financial and other incentives to optimize care. Setting up various reimbursement models, in combination with various practices, can help to determine what makes a significant difference in improving health care delivery (Stange et al., 2010, p. 606). All of these efforts are linked together by a better communications system that helps avoid unnecessary services, injuries that are medically induced (iatrogenic), and even broken appointments.

The person-centered medical home (PCHM) is now backed up by the group practices strong commitment to information technology and the use of data analysis to monitor patients with chronic diseases. There are now ways of employing electronic medical records to help families with members with chronic illness via reminders and prompts, according to personal health columnist Jane Brody (2010) as she lists the benefits of going digital.

> Improve care of chronic illnesses. Fewer than half of patients with chronic ailments regularly take prescribed medication or get the periodic checkups their doctors recommend. An electronic system can alert the physician to noncompliance and when it is time for another office visit. Electronic reminders and prompts can help patients get better preventive care . . ., like when they should have a colonoscopy, get a flu shot or get certain lab tests. Electronic records may also help to reduce waste in the system by identifying the most effective treatment regimens for common conditions. (p. D7)

The Pennsylvania program requires practices to meet standards set by the Washington DC–based National Committee on Quality Assurance (NCQA). This nonprofit organization is the child of the insurance industry and established three different levels of recognition for medical practices to meet to be financially rewarded by the participating health plans. Included are nine standards for performance, such as "adopts and implements evidence-based guidelines for three conditions."

It should come as no surprise that the insurance industry expects to realize huge savings from these efforts. The rewarding of physician practices for participation in the program that will lead to better care for people with chronic illnesses also aims to save insurance companies and public payers more than $1 billion that would be spent through hospital admissions during the three years of the Patient-Centered Primary Care Collaborative (2009).

Despite the promise of the Chronic Care Initiative, there are structural barriers to expansion of these programs so that people with chronic illnesses will receive the care they require to lead productive lives in the community. Enhancing primary care requires a financing structure that supports it; fee-for-service reimbursement does not, and in fact, it discourages the kind of reform of a disjointed delivery system that is found in most communities in the country (Baron and Cassel, 2008).

Related to the structural barriers imposed on primary care by the failure of the payment system to support it is the decline of the numbers of primary care providers in the United States, as noted by Richard J. Baron, one of the founders of Greenhouse Internists in Philadelphia, Pennsylvania, a forward-thinking collaborative. Baron (2009) notes that there is a chasm between intension and achievement in primary care because the labor supply is shrinking instead of increasing annually to meet the demand. General internists are leaving that practice within the first 10 years after completing training because they can make out better financially by becoming specialists in internal medicine. Given the burden of medical school debt, family medicine and ambulatory internal medicine is only chosen by approximately 1 out of 20 medical school graduates (Baron, 2009, p. 1922). Sadly, primary care, the centerpiece to health care reform, is not popular within the profession of medicine and this attitude is absorbed by the next generation of physicians.

Still, despite the shortages, some integrated health care organizations have had some success in making chronic care in the community pay off in terms of cost savings. Again the Keystone State supplies a case study of innovative health care through the Geisinger Health System. This integrated delivery system in central Pennsylvania employs 700 physicians in 55 clinical practice sites and runs three acute care hospitals, specialty hospitals, and ambulatory surgery facilities, which serve 215,000 covered lives in its health plan.

At all the Geisinger community sites, not just those that feature the PCMH, efforts are made to "provide a systematic approach to coordinated evidence-based care for patients with high-prevalence chronic diseases, including diabetes, congestive heart failure, chronic kidney disease, coronary artery disease, and hypertension" (Paulus, Davis, and Steele, 2008, p. 1240). Patients who are considered successfully tested and treated meet all the evidence-based care elements requirements. Those with known conditions when they enter the care system are tracked electronically to make sure that they receive all the tests required.

A multidisciplinary steering committee furnishes oversight on patient outcome goals, instructs on how to track patient progress, does financial analyses, negotiates payment terms with providers, and reviews insurance claims, program administration, and employer customer preferences (Paulus, Davis, and Steel, 2008). The result is that there is an ongoing and constant redesign effort that attempts to create adaptations to new knowledge so that care delivery does not lag behind. It is unlikely that community health centers devote as much time as the Geisinger system does to quality improvement, but there are several grades that the community health centers can achieve, and with improvement comes financial incentives to maintain high quality.

The Geisinger system also features a rapid response to delivery issues in its version of advanced primary care via the patient-centered medical home, called the "ProvenHealth Navigator." The development of this way of monitoring and improving the quality of care delivered was spurred by both the insurance and clinical side of this Quaker State Plan. At the start,

> this innovation addressed the fundamental needsof chronic disease patients with multiple conditions (for example, congestive heart failure, chronic obstructive pulmonary disease and diabetes) who represent the highest cost segment of our insurance company's membership. (Steele et al., 2010, p. 2048)

The takeaway for redesigning the delivery of services for quality improvement efforts at the Geisinger system was recognizing the limits of the stratification of patients by the level of acuity or severity would dictate how professional resources would be organized and distributed. The feedback of data from the insurance end of the plan, as well as study of patient-provider relationships, enabled the clinicians to make changes in the responsibilities shared by the care team. There were "new tasks for every member of the team, as well as new relationships between the on-site case management nurses and the primary care physician leader, between the primary care physician and the specialists; and between the primary care physician and post-acute care facilities and services" (Steele et al., 2010, p. 2051).

There were numerous adaptations performed to enhance the value of the care delivered. Care coordination services via nurses were available to all Medicaid patients during transition periods in the reengineered delivery system. Office staff and primary care physicians received training on how to perform acute-care management, using protocols and post-discharge templates that were created so that patients would be scheduled for appointments within three to five days of discharge. A greater emphasis on reporting was built on regular training sessions, including how to use trending graphs and perform utilization calculations. Physician leaders were made available for every four to six physicians so they could supply guidance. And finally, care coordination was enhanced through intensive discharge planning from nursing facilities to home (Steele et al., 2010, p. 2052).

All of this reorganization was backed up by new financial incentives generated by the insurance end of the operation. The planning process involved a review of the original program design and allowed for a refocusing on the needs of Medicare patients, independent of the level of severity.

The available evidence amassed by health delivery system experts from intensive literature reviews tends to support the initiatives to create both more providers to delivery primary care and to redirect primary care providers, and even specialists, to achieve such goals as lower rates of preventable hospitalization, emergency department visits, and lower mortality (Friedberg, Hussey, and Schneider, 2010, p. 769).

States that have more primary care physicians per capita are shown to have a healthier population and lower costs. Where specialists dominate, state medical spending per capita is higher and outcomes, quality of care, and patient satisfaction are no better than where there are fewer specialists relative to primary care providers (Bernstein, Chollet, Peikes, and Peterson, 2010, p. 1). In addition, where primary care initiatives have been attempted with Medicaid beneficiaries with one or more chronic conditions, as recently in Illinois, the success of the programs were attributed to primary care. The "Your Health Plus" and the "Illinois Health Connect" were medical home programs that delivered quality care and saved a total of $250 million a year in 2008 and 2009 (Arvantes, 2010).

Primary care is not just the foundation of improvements in quality in the United States but in other countries as well. As we have seen, Canada is starting to adopt the medical home model within its payment system. Europe is starting to recognize the value of primary care. Access to more primary care providers has been associated in Spain, as a result of a staggered remaking of the health care system, with reductions in hypertension and stroke-related mortality (Friedberg, Hussey, and Schneider, 2010, p. 769). The new bipartisan government in Great Britain, while it will not limit access to the National Health Service to reduce its enormous deficit, is seeking to use primary care doctors to avoid overreliance on specialty services, expensive technology, and hospital beds. While this reform sounds somewhat familiar, it is not being attempted in the United States while dealing with a shortage of primary care providers and creating insurance products for 37 million or more previously uncovered citizens and legally residing aliens. Despite these challenges, in the next chapter, I will review the current tools available in the United States to remake chronic care.

# 9

# Redesigning Health Care Delivery for the Age of Chronic Care

The Massachusetts health insurance reforms, first enacted in 2006, were clearly the model for the national health care reform bills introduced in both the House and the Senate in 2009 and finally signed by President Obama after a mighty struggle with conservative elements in the U.S. Congress in 2010. Making the process messy, a Republican strategy, did not keep the results from being regarded by many health policy commentators as a way to improve the quality of care for all while lowering the costs. The Republicans should note that most of the plan to extend insurance to the uninsured was created in one state, Massachusetts, under an extremely cooperative Republican with national ambitions, Governor Mitt Romney.

For the purposes of this chapter, two aspects of the Massachusetts experiment are worth noting. First, there is no difference in premiums for people with preexisting medical conditions so that even when a subscriber is a heavy user of services, the out-of-pocket costs to pay for the coverage will typically be no more than 7.5 to 10.6 percent of that person's income. Second, there is serious criticism of the Bay State plan from a health policy perspective because the coverage has made no difference in the delivery of medical services so that costs can be better contained (Steinbrook, 2008, p. 2760).

From the information on chronic conditions in the population collected by statewide health interview surveys, such as the one recently issued using 2007 data for Californians by the California Health Care Foundation, there is the clear possibility, through expanding primary care, to target and control chronic diseases with effective and regular outpatient care. Defining these conditions as manageable is the beginning of containment. Chronic illnesses, such as heart disease, cancer, stroke, or diabetes, are now called ambulatory care sensitive conditions (ACSCs) because they can be managed in the community, reducing the use of emergency department and hospital services as well as helping people with these conditions to live longer and have a better quality of life (Lui and Wallace, 2010).

The authors of this study, Lui and Wallace (2010, p. 3), also found that there was wide variation between counties in the Golden State with regard to the prevalence of various chronic diseases, both for adults and children. The proportion of adults reporting a chronic disease in affluent Marin County was 28 percent compared to almost 50 percent in what was designated the Tehama/Glenn/Colusa County cluster, a bastion of rural poverty. While the survey data in this statewide study concerning children did not show quite such high percentages having a chronic disease or being in poor health, there were still strong differences reported from the counties with the lowest percentages of these conditions versus those with the highest percentages. Reports by respondents on ease or difficulty in gaining access to care also varied by county. For the entire state, 25 percent of the adults with one or more chronic condition were also identified as having one or more barriers to health care use such as lack of health insurance, no usual source of care, and difficulty communicating with doctors. These barriers were associated with the acquisition of what are deemed preventable complications and avoidable hospitalizations (Lui and Wallace, 20010, p. 12). All of these results were based on a survey conducted during an affluent period and before the vast economic downturn shifted into full overdrive in 2008. Most states in 2009 reported sharply increased Medicaid enrollments, a result of people losing employer-based coverage or increasing financial inability to afford to continue to pay premiums, including those with chronic illnesses, leading to the introduction of the redirection of the financing of the care system to make the state dollars go further and maximize the federal contribution. Medicaid is designed to expand counter-cyclically, but this latest and greatest recession is emptying out state treasuries, even when there are increases in funding from the federal government's stimulus package. Federal aid to states to sustain Medicaid was passed in August 2010, a time when many states were facing enormous state deficits that could not constitutionally be addressed by issuing bonds since this mechanism for raising money can only be used to pay for capital projects such as building bridges, roads and tunnels, or college dormitories.

Some health delivery system planners have started to introduce the idea that getting better value for the Medicaid dollars is a good idea. There is a need to get the Medicaid expenditures to purchase better results in health care delivery to the poor and disabled. The desire on the part of health policy wonks to redesign the delivery system to address the needs of healthy patients and those with chronic diseases by permitting them greater access to primary care and specialty care that is delivered through ambulatory care clinics has led some states to rethink the payment system to Medicaid providers so that funds are shifted from inpatient care to outpatient care services. These financial incentives are regarded as initiatives to get better value for the money spent on facilities and staff, assuming that academic medical centers and government-run hospitals can make a successful transformation happen. With Medicaid enrollments rising in every state due to the economic downturn, this kind of realignment of services would make sense, as office-based fee schedules rise, at least in New York State to 72 percent of Medicare rates while facility rates rise only to 56 percent of Medicare (Bachrach, 2009).

The idea of getting better value for the funds that are distributed to providers in the financing of health care does not stop with Medicaid. Increasingly, there is an attempt to prioritize the application of a methodology of what is known about how to get better results in health care, especially when it comes to the delivery of chronic care. Improving patient outcomes has become part of a more patient-oriented and more goal-oriented approach to the delivery system. The patient-centered medical home is evaluated not just on how much it humanizes the transactions between consumers and providers but also with regard to the extent to which clinical performance is improving patient outcomes. Medical groups and other organizations in health care, according to some advocates for change, need to be evaluated on whether or not the care they deliver gets good results (Bohmer and Lee, 2009, p. 1347). Even insurers, such as Empire Blue Cross and Blue Shield of New York, are starting to look for improvements of outcomes when it comes to setting rates with hospitals and medical centers now that the means to measure them reliably are available.

The providers such as medical groups and hospitals are willing, for example, to offer follow-up care for a patient discharged from a hospital following treatment for congestive heart failure, but they may not reap the financial benefits from offering post-hospital care. Hospital administrators have hardly fought hard to get the idea of the bundled payment into the health care reform legislation since saving money on the cost of hospital stays only goes to the payer and not the provider, yet incentives can be created to give hospitals a stake in the new game. The business side of the equation needs to be considered when the redesign of services takes place, allowing for a win-win situation for Medicare, for example, and major medical centers that utilize their resources far beyond payment to reduce readmissions (Abelson, 2009).

There are other issues related to consumer cooperation that require some new ways for physicians to relate to their patients. Incentives in the new health care reform legislation will help motivate physicians to move in this direction. However, some patients may be reluctant to get their care at home and through ambulatory care visits to their general internal medicine clinicians. Getting the physicians on board to purchase better health care at lower cost for people with chronic illnesses means that they have to believe in what they do. The public when becoming patients can be concerned about innovations to improve chronic care since they have not become familiar with these new ways of doing things.

A radio story from the Bay Area of California's public radio station, KQED, points to the skepticism often expressed by patients about whether a primary care physician can coordinate and treat the medical problems of a patient with diabetes, rather than requiring an encounter with a subspecialist such as an endocrinologist (Varney, 2010). The Geisinger Health System, previously discussed with regard to the idea of the patient-centered medical home, was also the subject of a popular article in the "Your Health" section of the Association of American Retired Persons (AARP) April 2009 *Bulletin* that focused on the need to change attitudes, often derived from patients' experiences with the silos of the delivery system.

Delivery system reform has to accompany the reform of financing and the introduction of consumer protections that will come from the Affordable Care Act, according to Paul Ginsburg, president of the Center for Studying Health System Change, a nonprofit organization that focuses on how to spend the health care dollar more wisely (Barry, 2009, p. 12). The Geisinger system not only attempted to get the doctors in rural Pennsylvania to convince their patients that the patient-centered medical home would allow them to stay out of the hospital and lead richer lives, but it also adopted the checklist approach on how to prepare for surgical procedures (Barry, 2009, p. 14).

The simple but methodical use of the checklist approach, advocated widely by the surgeon and the qualitatively oriented health systems expert Atul Giwande, is also compatible with the awesome techno-logical advancements in surgery such as robotics. But we also need to dig more deeply in trying to find out how to create a high-quality health care system for people with chronic conditions. Robert H. Brook (2009), in writing about the science of health care reform, raised an important question in the social engineering of the future: "How can physicians change the health care system in ways that both are sensitive to the needs of individual patients and reflect population level data?" (p. 2487).

Brook (2009) then proceeds to focus on assessing the appropriate-ness of performing a procedure on a patient, the need for reliable information to make that assessment, the barriers to eliminating unnecessary medical and surgical procedures, and the extent to which simple procedures that are safe and inexpensive can substitute for big ticket interventions. Brook is looking for ways to compare results so that systemic change will come; and we are at a point in the history of medicine where we can say that there are ways to accomplish this goal. Clearly, comparative effectiveness research, a designation for efforts to find out which diagnostic techniques and clinical interventions work best and at what cost, must be a major component of any new efforts to redesign the way chronic care, which accounts for 70 percent of health expenditures in the United States, is delivered.

While not exactly the most popular subject on network television, or even subscription stations on cable, comparative effectiveness research was supported strongly in the Obama administration's 2009 stimulus bill (ARRA) to the tune of $1.1 billion to put in place a mecha-nism to slow health care spending, especially where chronic care is concerned. It also is a powerful alternative to rationing care according to the capacity of the patient to benefit from it. It is one way to help shrink a bloated and, at times, ineffective health care system. And this approach has support from some veterans of the efforts to reduce pub-lic expenditures on health care. Gail Wilensky (2009), a former Bush 41 administrator of the Health Care Finance Administration, the prede-cessor agency to the Centers for Medicare and Medicaid Services, has identified the various stakeholders who may support or object to findings generated by a federal center on comparative effectiveness research, suggesting that the progress in bending the curve of health care expenditures may not be all that simple once the facts are known. Yet she concedes that

Comparative effectiveness research combined with changes in reimbursement that reward and encourage the use of the most clinically appropriate and valuable interventions can help slow health spending while maintaining incentives for valuable medical innovation.

Avatars, to borrow a name from contemporary popular culture, for comparative effectiveness research have challenged contemporary medical practice to reduce the waste in the health care system by avoiding what they designate as "marginal medicine" (Hoffman and Pearson, 2009). What this characterization boils down to are four evidence-related categories of practices that yield little in the way of value for the patient (p. w712–13).

- Inadequate evidence of comparative net benefit, given the risks
- Use beyond boundaries of the established net benefit, meaning uncertainty regarding interventions, including drugs where there is no evidence of a net benefit
- Higher cost when net benefit is comparable to other options rather than being clearly superior
- Relatively high cost for incremental benefit compared to other options, meaning that minimal advantages and costs judged to be too high should place an intervention in the category of marginal medicine

Comparative effectiveness research, while restricted in scope in the Affordable Care Act to avoid any hint of rationing, or more popularly, "pulling the plug on Grandma," will have an impact by furnishing information to decision makers as to what treatments give the best bang for the buck. A health policy brief issued by *Health Affairs* and the Robert Wood Johnson Foundation in late 2010 concludes that value-based health requires this kind of information.

> If there is more clarity about which treatments work best—and for which patients—there's potential for shifting money to those interventions and stay away from less effective treatments. (Health Policy Brief, 2010, p. 4)

A great deal of this kind of valuable research, moving forward, will be based on the availability of information about patient visits to health care providers, the test results from wherever the tests were performed, and authorization from the patient that this information can not only be shared among the various specialists and primary care practitioners visited but also can be put into a large database to determine the effectiveness of various interventions. Clinical researchers will be able to make sharper distinctions between what works and what does not with larger samples of patients seen in a variety of settings. Some of these opportunities for decisive research depend on the proliferation of patient-controlled medical records across numerous academic medical centers, and in so doing, making location at one academic medical center or another unimportant as long as data are available. As one team of authors sees it in a lyrical fashion:

> This scenario anticipates a new scale of data liquidity, a gush of information from clinical settings—electronic health records, laboratory information systems, and medication-management systems into PCHR platforms where health care consumers independently decide about subsequent disclosures. (Mandl and Kohane, 2008, p. 1730)

While the day when this kind of easy transfer and use of clinical information may still be sometime into the future, there is great potential for using it to benefit patients in the daily practice of health care delivery, especially with patients receiving chronic care in a medical home.

Research on how to reduce hospital readmission rates, using the electronic medical record, may go far beyond simply realigning incentives between the medical center and the doctor who must keep the patient from returning to the hospital bed. Once alignments are in place, there is still the task of determining which practices among hospital personnel and primary care physicians prevent readmissions and which do not. Sometimes comparisons of different rates of home visits for patients with similar chronic diseases, for example, can show benefits of four visits per month by the nurse practitioner rather than two a month. Alternatively, it might happen that two visits are just as good as four and allows the nurse practitioner to have a bigger case load.

Keeping people with chronic diseases out of the hospital via the appropriate use of the patient-centered medical home can reduce expenditures and limit patient exposure to diseases picked up in the hospital, technically designated as nosocomial illnesses. Risk-adjusted readmission rates can be compared and provider variables introduced as independent variables to see what predicts effective care. Patient discharge planning, done in a comprehensive fashion, has already been shown in a meta-analysis of 18 studies in eight countries to reduce readmission rates, as discussed by Arnold Epstein (2009) in an essay about shared accountability (p. 1458).

The professional associations with a stake in ambulatory care are also pushing for more study of what works. There is a robust research agenda being developed through the collaboration of the major physician-oriented academic primary care societies, the Society of

General Internal Medicine, the Society of Teachers of Family Medicine, and the Academic Pediatric Association. The agenda is patient focused within the context of the patient-centered medical home (PCMH).

> Measuring patient-centeredness as a PCMH outcome requires patient surveys that directly assess the extent to which patients' needs and desires are met, their concerns are addressed and they feel adequately engaged and able to provide input into both their personal health care decisions and the practice organization. (Rittenhouse, Thom, and Schmittdiel, 2010, p. 594)

Process is important when you want patients to take ownership for their care. Patients, therefore, are surveyed to find out if they were part of the development of the treatment plan, whether there were choices made within the plan, that it could be carried out in their daily lives, and that their beliefs, values, and traditions were taken into account when treatments were recommended. This kind of information collection has its roots in the patient satisfaction surveys that were started by John Ware in the 1960s as part of the public evaluation of Medicare, allowing the backers of this public health insurance program to say that the receivers of health care services paid for by Medicare were pleased with what they got and they did not feel like second-class citizens or welfare recipients, as some critics of the program suggested would happen.

Measurement does not end with the patient's satisfaction but also seeks to determine the impact of the PCMH on the outcomes of care, including good chronic disease management to reduce the incidence of complications that can produce emergency visits or hospitalization for diabetic flare-ups and other primary care sensitive conditions (PCS). Early readmissions for PCS conditions such as congestive heart failure or chronic lung disease are considered indicators of avoidable hospitalizations because they are ambulatory care sensitive.

Primary care providers led the way in making Grand Junction, Colorado, a leader in good outcomes, one of the most ambulatory care sensitive health care regions as well as reducing per capita spending for Medicare patients to 24 percent of the national average. As mentioned in the Preface, the success of this effort captured national attention and a visit by President Obama. Moreover, in this city of 50,000 residents, the Rocky Mountain Health Plans, or Rocky, and the Mesa County Physicians Independent Practice Association (MCPIPA), through the advocacy and deal-making work of family physicians, created a payment system where there was equal payment to doctors regardless of whether the patient was covered by Medicaid, Medicare, or private insurance. Under these conditions of practice, "in 2006, Grand Junction had 85% more family doctors per capita than the national average" (Bodenheimer and West, 2010, p. 1392). And with doctors receiving a set fee for each patient seen in their practices, making access to primary care for Medicaid patients less burdensome, there was a reduction in the use of the emergency department. Consequently, there was a "low per-enrollee cost for Medicaid acute care" (Bodenheimer and West, 2010, p. 1392).

The incentive system at the independent practice association in Grand Junction also included a reserve fund of 15 percent of patient fees that was distributed to the participating primary and specialty care physicians if costs were controlled for the year. In addition, specialists whose rates of performing expensive procedures, such as cardiac catheterizations were out of line with other cardiologists, were identified publicly in the medical community and were encouraged to change their practice style. (No further public humiliations took place.) Primary care physicians subtly let specialists who were performing unnecessary interventions know, via restricting referrals to those outliers, that their practice styles would not be tolerated.

An important feature of this story about the town that bent the cost curve had to do with restricted resources in Grand Junction; since there was only one tertiary care hospital in town, there was limited access to operating rooms and hospital beds that involved expensive interventional cardiac and neurosurgery procedures (Bodenheimer and West, 2010, p. 1393). It has often been noted that communities with excess hospital beds per capita often experience more surgeries and other kinds of hospital admissions. While every locality furnishes different conditions, leadership by the primary care community can be a way to take up this model of development and gain better outcomes while lowering health care expenditures. The methodology of how they got to be delivering quality services at modest cost needs to be disseminated widely and scaled up.

Perhaps the most impressive scaled-up efforts at avoiding hospitalizations is found in the previously discussed Geisinger Health System, based in Danville, Pennsylvania, a fully integrated system employing 800 physicians in 43 counties and serving a population of 2.6 million, with 500,000 active patients (Dentzer, 2010c, p. 1200). Thirty percent of the patients are insured by Geisinger, affording this system an opportunity to take risks with innovations. Under the leadership of Glenn Steele, MD, the Geisinger system has developed an advanced medical home for chronic disease care optimization (ProvenHealth Navigator). As Steele reveals in an interview with the editor of *Health Affairs*, the program is constantly being reengineered.

> We changed the incentives for our physicians, on the primary care side as well as on the specialty side. We put insurance company-employed nurses in the primary care practices and even in the skilled nursing facilities where many of our patients were living.
>
> The fact of the matter is, we're keeping these patients healthier, so that even with their multiple chronic diseases, they don't end up in emergency rooms at 10:00 p.m. on Friday night with shortness of breath, seeking a well-meaning emergency doctor they've never seen before, who cannot get to their records, and being admitted for a "tune up." That's kind of an encapsulated view of what happens to a lot of patients with multiple chronic diseases, and it happens to them over and over again. (Dentzer, 2010c, p. 1204)

The advanced form of the medical home, another name for the PCMH, used by the Geisinger system, has produced sharply reduced rates of readmissions for the 65,000 patients who receive these services. These results are based on rewards and planning. Not only are primary care physicians paid via cross-subsidies a great deal more than other PCPs in the 43 counties covered by the Geisinger system, but there is a strong emphasis on employing nurse practitioners, physician assistants, and other physician extenders embedded in the community and, again, paid for by the Geisinger insurance company. According to Steele,

> Nurses were essentially the 24/7 triage person responsible for everything that happened to 125–150 patients. They provided concierge care for the sickest, not concierge care for the richest. If the patient needed to see the primary care physician who was the head of the team, they were. If they needed to be seen by the specialist, they were. But the general contractor in charge of the triage was the nurse. (Dentzer, 2010c, p. 1206)

Success seemed to breed success, with the Geisinger nurses starting to create innovations in a practice that went beyond the high utilizing patients, e.g., those with congestive heart failure, but armed with insurance company data, they saw that there was unjustified variation in the quality of care and outcomes with regard to other subpopulations, and they went after them as well.

As one might anticipate, the difficult cases are not based on patients with a single chronic disease, no matter how much a patient with congestive heart failure will require in the form of maintenance, but reside with patients with multiple chronic conditions. Boult and

Wieland (2010), in a series in the *Journal of the American Medical Association* on "care of the aging patient: from evidence to action," offers both a case study of how advanced primary care should be planned and delivered for a patient with "a history of hypertension with left ventricular hypertrophy, peripheral vascular disease, with a left below the knee amputation, chronic obstructive pulmonary disease (COPD), glaucoma, keratitis, osteoarthritis with chronic right should pain, and degenerative intervertebral disk disease" (p. 1936). The intervention for Ms. N was based on four concurrent and interacting processes summarized below, including:

• Comprehensive assessment, including diseases, disabilities, medications, personal capacities, preferences, and community supports
• Creation, implementation, and monitoring of a evidence-based plan of care
• Communication and coordination with all who provide care for the patient
• Involvement of the patient (and caregiver) in his or her health care

The availability of these four processes is rare in ordinary primary care where few physicians are trained to engage in team approaches to patient care. Prior to being admitted to a local Program of All-Inclusive Care for the Elderly (PACE), Ms. N's condition continued to deteriorate and she was in and out of hospitals and skilled nursing facilities. PACE patients are living in the community but certified by the state as eligible for nursing facility care; by virtue of the skilled and coordinated care she received, Ms. N's chronic conditions became more manageable, her health status improved, and she demonstrated greater self-sufficiency during the six years that she was followed by the program's staff physicians.

The authors not only did a case study but also did a structural comparison of PACE to two other programs that are similar in approach, the Geriatric Resources for Assessment and Care of Elders (GRACE) and Guided Care, but that utilized the patient's original primary care physician (PCP) as the center of the medical home. Despite the promise of reinventing primary care to fit the chronic care model, it is not at all certain that most PCPs want to remake their practices into patient-centered medical homes and/or join accountable care organizations to participate in the delivery of financially well-aligned and thereby cost-effective services to patients with multiple chronic illnesses (Boult and Wieland, 2010).

Finally, strictly from a cost perspective, there have been some insurance plans that have created products for group policies wherein they develop physician profiles so they classify those doctors who offer less-expensive care. These products suggest that the same quality of care can be received from providers who are more conservative in their resource utilization than others, thereby helping patients while lowering their out-of-pocket costs. While it is difficult to determine whether generalists are better at cost containment than specialists, some health delivery researchers have already concluded that the methods used for profiling physicians with respect to cost of services can generate misleading results (Adams, Mehrotra, Thomas, and McGlynn, 2010). These are important issues to address in the critical implementation and regulation writing stages of the key provisions of the Affordable Care Act, a subject that will be debated among various camps of researchers who study the health care delivery and financing systems. Central to the success of the Affordable Care Act is the sufficient funding for the Department of Health and Human Services (HHS) during regulation writing and implementation time so that appropriate staffing for these tasks can take place. The continuing resolutions that Congress has passed in 2010 suggest that requested funding for expanding the capacity of HHS has not taken place to permit on-time regulation writing and implementation of the ACA. The results are going to lay out the course of growth and value-oriented innovations in health care in America, largely affecting older Americans. Meanwhile, as an aging American, this old codger, with the help of learned optimism, will explain in the final chapter how the Affordable Care Act will promote better chronic care, despite the potential shortage of primary care providers.

# 10

# The Reach of the 2010 Affordable Care Act: Implications for Chronic Care

On March 23, 2010, President Barack Obama signed into law the Health Care and Education Affordability Reconciliation Act of 2010 (HR 4872), a major remedy for the health care insecurity that plagued many Americans without insurance coverage because of the cost of premiums and often their rejection from commercial insurance policies because of preexisting conditions. This was clearly a milestone in a number of ways.

- For individuals with chronic conditions, who make up the entire population of those who either cannot afford insurance because the premiums are "experience rated" and therefore based on anticipation of potential policyholders making a disproportionate number of claims, or because the insurance companies would not underwrite them no matter what the cost, this shameful chapter in U.S. history came to an end and a new era of greater fairness began.
- For many of the think tanks around the country who provided the guidance for the development of the statutes that became part of what is now called the Affordable Care Act, this was a time for celebration and vindication. The Robert Wood Johnson Foundation, in particular, built on the work of Ed Wagner and created the Chronic Care Model that became the centerpiece of the Foundation's national program—*Improving Chronic Illness Care*.
- And, later, for many of the advance practice nurses and other health practitioners, the Act would be an opportunity to create the capacity to do chronic care as well as other aspects of primary care. So when on August 5, 2010, Health and Human Services Secretary Kathleen Sebelius announced that more than $159 million would go for training geriatric care workers, there was further celebration at the education programs that train nurses and geriatric specialists. (Aizenman, 2010)

In the signing ceremony, President Obama not only took note of the fact that the reforms found in the Affordable Care Act (ACA) were as important as the introduction of Medicare and Medicaid in 1965, but that it strongly represented "the core principle that everybody should have some basic security when it comes to their health care." Many advocates of universal coverage, including myself, would have preferred the nationalization of the financing of health care insurance through what is called a single payer system, modeled after the program adopted by Canada more than 35 years ago and not that different from what is in place in most advanced industrial societies such as Japan, France, and Germany. An extension of Medicare to the entire population, a 45-year-old program that has made a huge difference in the lives of the elderly and people with disabilities, could mean basically that we adopt a single payer financing system. Covering everyone would not be driven by the controversial individual mandate since premiums would be paid for through payroll taxes, a form of social insurance, and supplemented by funds from general federal taxation to cover those who are too poor or unemployed and therefore would not support FICA, or the Federal Insurance Corporation of America payments for Social Security and Medicare.

While the president was eloquent, as usual, on signing day, he did not mention that health care reform goes beyond individual security from medical debt and bankruptcy. The country has to prepare for the enormous shift in demographics, already noted in the 2010 census report, one which will mean that given the huge increase in the population 65 and over in 2030, that we need to determine how this group, with their disproportionate numbers and with several chronic illnesses, is going to be given medical care without bankrupting the federal government and allowing those who need care coordination a chance to lead independent lives.

The answer largely lies in transforming the health care system to scale-up care coordination so that it is a hybrid delivery system that can be defined as a "person centered, assessment-based interdisciplinary approach to integrating health care and social support services in which a care coordinator manages and monitors an individual's needs, goals and preferences based on a comprehensive plan" (Berenson and Howell, 2009, p. 2).

Coordinated care requires some sophisticated alignments of different parts of the existing health care system, including private insurance, if is going to make a difference both globally and individually as we move forward. One skeptic, Jeff Goldsmith (2010, p. 1302), argues that the concept of chronic care coordination involves so many providers, state-of-the-art information technology, and multiple steps to take that it is only possible to do it well in large group practices or hospital systems, similar to Geisinger System of Pennsylvania. Nevertheless, systems can be cobbled together from smaller units, a strategy we are likely to see in the future.

The ACA did not go as far as I would like in covering everyone at a reasonable price. What did finally become law fell short of what more decisive reform would entail while still maintaining for-profit insurance companies. This was a deliberate decision on the part of the Obama team, despite pressure from the Left to move more in the direction of classical social insurance. Even in the course of the development of this bill, progressives advocated the inclusion of a vigorous or robust public option to be upheld as a benchmark for insurance companies so that they would pay more attention to serving their beneficiaries than to realizing profits. The hope was that the public option would woo most Americans without insurance away from the commercial product to one that was able to offer coverage at lower cost, was willing to deal fairly with policyholders, and perhaps would even offer more benefits.

Keeping costs down from the liberal or progressive perspective focused mostly on the profits and administrative expenses of the health insurance giants of the United States. Additionally, we progressives also advocated that the re-importation of pharmaceuticals should be permitted in the United States so that consumers could get the same discounts that Canadians or citizens of other countries received from the manufacturers of the drugs that extend life and improve the quality of living for many of us, especially senior citizens. Why should Americans alone bear the price of research, discovery, and formulation of new pharmaceuticals? Additionally, we advocated that the Medicare Part D drug program be allowed to negotiate with the pharmaceutical manufacturers to receive discounted prices on brand names and to shorten the period of patent protection for them so that generic drugs could be acquired at more reasonable costs in a shorter wait time. For many of the critics of the health care legislation from the perspective of advocates of a social insurance approach, we were able to get over our disappointment and accept the half loaf that was proffered. Nevertheless, single payer will not go away and some national organizations are still keeping hope alive. Despite these organizations to the left of the president, the Republicans continue to call the Affordable Care Act "socialized medicine" and talked about repealing it during the run-up to the 2010 election. How could this be "socialized medicine" when health providers remain independent under the ACA; doctors are not employees of the government and hospitals are not owned by the nation or individual states; payment for care does not come only from taxation, a dedicated payroll tax, or some combination of the two sources of revenue? There is a long way to go before the United States has "socialized medicine," although Medicare and Medicaid are both wildly popular among recipients.

Despite the absence of these reform measures, such as the public option, from the final legislation, there is much to be proud of in the effort to end some of the inequities in health care due to the insurance industry's transparent strategy of risk avoidance and therefore keeping the medical-loss ratio as high as possible. Clearly, following a period of transition, there will be opportunity for the uninsured to gain control over their health care coverage; older people (among them those with known chronic conditions) will be able to purchase insurance from an exchange at a price that may not be the same as that offered to younger individuals, but will be no more than 300 percent of the strict community rate. To maintain a fair system of charges, rates will be based on age rather than health conditions. Moreover, those with preexisting conditions will be eligible, as early as August 2010 in some states, for subsidized coverage through a nationally financed high-risk pool. If a person is denied coverage because of a preexisting condition and has been without insurance for six months, confirming that he or she did not simply drop coverage, that person will qualify for the state risk pool, scheduled to be up and running, as planned, 90 days after the signing of the ACA. If states decline to develop the risk pool, HHS will step in and do it.

There are other advantages in the new legislation for people with chronic illnesses. For those who acquire serious chronic illnesses while in a plan, insurance companies will be prohibited from revoking coverage for those who get sick. In addition, insurance companies will no longer be permitted to set lifetime limits on indemnifying a beneficiary or restricting benefits to cover needed medical procedures (Davis and Collins, 2010). Young adults, up to the age of 26, will be able to remain on their parents' health care policies, getting close to some of the insurance laws of the progressive states that require coverage up to the age of 31. For young adults with serious chronic illnesses, continuity in coverage is vital to their quality of life. Finally, children with serious chronic illnesses will no longer be taken off their parents' policies or only covered for health care outside of the disease that requires a great deal of attention.

## REALIGNING INCENTIVES TO PROVIDERS

There is attention paid to the need to realign the incentives to professionals and organizations in the health care delivery system as well as create security for consumers. The new law has a plan to reduce expenditures driven by health care providers looking out for their financial solvency and not the patient's best interest. Most importantly, there are funds available through the Affordable Care Act to establish incentives to providers to reduce unnecessary hospitalizations. Many of the ideas expressed in the early chapters of this book are now accepted as in a final review stage or are considered state-of-the art practices. Through the newly created Center for Medicare and Medicaid Innovation, the impact of new methods of payment such as bundled payments for hospital, accountable care organizations, and post-acute care will be evaluated. In addition, incentives for establishing and expanding medical homes and accountable care organizations will also be fostered by this new branch of the Center for Medicare and Medicaid Services (Davis and Collins, 2010). Doctors will be given financial incentives to join accountable care organizations and hospitals will similarly be incentivized to reduce readmissions due to preventable causes such as infections (Medicare Rights Center, 2010).

But it will take more than simply offering financial incentives or bundling payments. There is clearly a requirement for new forms of organizing doctors and hospitals into caregiving entities that all buy into. This is not easy to accomplish, given that the threat to existing financing means a threat to stability and medical care as we know it. The New York State Health Foundation (2010) has recognized that the acceptance of a new alignment of incentives that would promote bundled payments is not simply doing the math.

> hospitals, physicians and other post-acute providers will need to organize into networks capable of sharing payments and adhering to uniform policies and procedures. Unless financial relationships already exist, this is expected to be particularly difficult to implement. Throughout the process of designing and implementing a bundled payment methodology, all stakeholders will need to be sure to avoid any restrictions imposed by antitrust requirements. (p. 3)

Physicians and advance practice nurses will receive financial incentives to create better forms of chronic care coordination via funds available through the new law. Unquestionably, primary care has to be greatly expanded through Medicaid to accommodate the newly entitled eligible people at 133 percent of poverty. In 2013 and 2014, states will be financed for several years with 100 percent federal funding, or close to it, to pay for the services required as Medicaid takes in more individuals. A significant part of this population needs chronic care, often unavailable when they were not covered by Medicaid. The delivery system has to be readied for this influx of vulnerable people. This increase in covered lives via Medicaid, a federal-state program, will put strains on the health delivery system. To motivate physicians such as family physicians, general internists, and general pediatricians, the Affordable Care Act mandates that primary care physicians be compensated at the rate that Medicare pays for primary care. This should make medical care more accessible to individuals with chronic illnesses as well as those who are healthy. The proliferation of effective accountable care organizations depends on the alignment of incentives for doctors to join and coordinate care from specialists as well as improve patient health. To reduce the unnecessary readmission to hospitals of patients with multiple chronic illnesses, especially those who are Medicare recipients, requires this kind of reorganization and refinancing of chronic care.

## HELP WITH THE COST OF PRESCRIPTION MEDICATIONS

For many of us who dwell, by dint of age, in the Lipitor nation, staying well or deteriorating slowly requires daily maintenance doses of powerful but expensive medications, although generics are now available to replace Lipitor at a great savings to the payer, whether a pharmacy plan or the individual. Health insecurity persists for those seniors and people deemed disabled, whose income and assets do not allow them to be eligible for both Medicare and Medicaid. The high cost of medications for people of moderate or low income is a serious problem and is also being tackled by health care reform. Much of chronic care is built around access to medications, which can put the user in a deep hole financially. Pharmacy benefits, Medicare Part D, a recent addition to Medicare, 2006, are noticeably underfunded by this plan for assistance and available for those who have limited expenses for medications (a sop to the majority of seniors so they would support Medicare expansion) and those who have catastrophic expenses that could, if not covered, lead to losing one's home to pay for drugs. Those in the middle remain vulnerable and this needed a correction.

One of the most significant changes from the perspective of people who require chronic care is the change in Medicare Part D—the gradual closing of what is known as the donut hole. Quickly, currently those who are signed up for Part D receive assistance for the first $3,599 of prescription expenses and must pay 100 percent of the next $2,500 of expenses, before they again receive assistance with their drug bills. While closure of the gap will be gradual, it means that Medicare eligible individuals who have reached the amount of $3,600 in prescription expenditures receive, starting in 2010, a $250 rebate but still be, as they are now, required to pay full price for pharmaceuticals. Starting in 2011, those in the donut hole will receive a 50 percent discount on brand name drugs, with a progressive decrease in the share of expenses accumulated in this gap in coverage until it returns to the standard 25 percent for the rest of the Part D plan (Medicare Rights Center, 2010).

## MEASURING CLINICAL EFFECTIVENESS

There is also another major initiative that is worth discussing from the perspective of a person with a chronic illness, or indeed from the viewpoint of anyone who might have to take medication or undergo a medical procedure. The nonprofit Patient Centered Outcomes Research Institute will evaluate existing research and conduct studies to find out about the "relative health outcomes, clinical effectiveness and appropriateness" of different medical treatments (Kaiser Health News Staff, 2010). Despite the fear of a "government takeover" regarding what will be permitted, the findings regarding therapeutic effectiveness will hardly be rammed down the throats of patients with chronic illnesses. Scaremongering has not diminished now that the ACA is the law of the land. No part of the Affordable Care Act, when it was being debated, was more subject to outrageous and lying interpretations than the section on the "heartless agency" that was going to use these findings to deny care to the elderly or people with chronic care needs. The demagogues on the Right were successful in getting stripped out of the bill any support for end-of-life discussions between doctors and their patients and paid for by Medicare but the idea of clinical effectiveness research prevailed with several restraints in place.

First, patient-centered outcomes research will be filtered by a directorship recruited from various stakeholders. The institute will be run by a governing board of 19 members, including patients, doctors, hospitals, drug makers, device manufacturers, payers, government officials, and health experts. The work of the institute will only be advisory through information to the health care industry, professionals, and consumers. It will take time to accept the recommendations of the research team at the institute.

Second, this institute was designed to use the power of persuasion, not legal authority, to implement restrictions on clinical care. It will not have the power to require or demonstrate approval for changes or elimination of a particular treatment. Nor can it introduce a procedure that is brand new and with which the medical community is not familiar.

There are also some benchmarks established for measuring patient-centered care that can help determine what is and what is not patient-centered care. According to Epstein, Fiscella, Lesser, and Stange (2010), and supported by all family medicine experts from the halls of academe, journals, and foundations, there is in place a way to determine if patient-centered care is going forward.

> A recent National Cancer Institute monograph outlines six measurable aspects of patient-centered care: fostering healing relationships, exchanging information, responding to emotions, managing uncertainty, making decisions, and enabling self-management. (p. 1493)

These social features may be a way of certifying programs that will receive funding for furnishing appropriate services, a way to make sure that Medicare and other insurers will get value for their payments.

Third, the institute will have more command as to what Medicare will pay for. The Kaiser Health News writers (2010) indicate that "Medicare may take the Institute's research into account when deciding what procedures it will cover, so long as the new research is not the sole justification and the agency allows for public input." In other words, the cold hand of science will be tempered by allowing the warm and fuzzy nonresearch community to have its say.

## MEDICARE SHARED SAVINGS PROGRAM

The elements of the Medicare Shared Savings Program define what is known in health reform circles as the accountable care organization (ACO). It is designed to scale-up from the pilot programs described earlier in this treatise, to allow for more robust demonstration projects. When formed by health care providers, the ACO becomes accountable for "the quality, cost, and overall care of the Medicare fee-for-service beneficiaries assigned to it" (HR 3590, 2010, p. 730). An ACO has to be staffed with primary care professionals in sufficient numbers to provide the care required for 5,000 beneficiaries. Note that the language does not say that these professionals all have to be medical doctors. This opens the door for nurse practitioners, despite their limited numbers, to ply their craft as well as family physicians, general pediatricians, and general internists.

Technologies that are state-of-the-art in distance delivery of services will be utilized to promote evidence-based medicine and patient involvement. Advanced techniques such as telehealth, a form of remote patient monitoring, will expand the reach of the primary care provider (HR 3590, 2010, p. 731). Moreover, a strong emphasis on measurement of the quality of care through process and outcome measures will be part of the evaluation process. To promote transparency, data will be submitted to the Center on Medicare and Medicaid Services (CMS) to see whether these demonstration programs meet quality performance standards. Reporting requirements will be linked to incentive payments under another part of the law, section 1848, entitled the physician quality reporting initiative (PQRI).

Safeguards are included to prevent ACOs that receive bundled payments for fee-for-service Medicare beneficiaries to furnish all the care required, as well as reduce costs, without avoiding the more expensive-to-serve patients. In other words, the fine art of "cherry picking," learned from the way insurance companies avoid risk, will be watched carefully by the CMS and high-maintenance patients will have to be included among those served. Where appropriate, the programs that skim the cream, so to speak, will be subject to sanctions (HR 3590, 2010, p. 737).

Some provider organizations are getting in on the action early. In the spring of 2010, nationally, a consortium of 2,300 hospitals, going under the name Premier, launched a new venture in accountable care. Nineteen new accountable care organizations (ACO) will furnish care for 1.2 million patients, based on a partnership with 70 hospitals and 5,000 physicians. This is no pilot project but a permanent effort, complete with a "shared savings model" that will make it possible for hospitals to benefit from not admitting patients (Reichard, 2010b). This could be the beginning of the end of silos!

Premier will continue to recruit hospital systems and doctors through a program that screens for readiness to collaborate. In finding programs that are ready, the organizers are looking for skills, team, and operational capabilities that establish the capacity to become ACOs. Some of the funding will come from Medicare under the Affordable Care Act and the collaboratives will also attempt to enlist other payers (insurers) who are interested in keeping patients healthy through coordinated primary care (Reichard, 2010b). Growing the program is essential for gaining acceptance in the health care field as well as for scaling-up.

Despite my enthusiasm for the collaboratives, the big uncertainty that remains with regard to ACOs has to do with incentives for hospitals and specialists—will ACOs be large enough to entice them to participate? For some chief executive officers who have been successful at running the functional equivalent of an ACO, such as my colleague, Steven Safyer, MD, at Montefiore Medical Center in the Bronx, governance is key. In other words, the form of payment to doctors at this academic linked health care facility, dedicated to serving the urban poor and nonpoor, is based on salaries, and there is no incentive to specialists or primary care providers to do extra procedures to generate personal income as in a straight fee-for-service payment reward system. In addition, the governance plan of Montefiore Medical Center allows funds to be moved to where they are needed and not remain in silos to be managed or distributed by the units that helped accumulate these funds.

Experts on health care reform also note emphatically that health insurance reform is not going to reduce costs unless it is accompanied by the emergence of new delivery system models that can alter provider practices that seem to be cast in stone. ACOs, if they have sufficient size and scope, can deliver services to a large part of the population, including people in need of chronic care. Organizations that step forward to become ACOs for assigned Medicare beneficiaries have to be willing to be responsible for care at the per capita payments they receive. While they may legally get to keep the savings rendered, they are also held accountable for cost overruns. Saving can be used as a reserve to take care of the expenses that cannot be paid for from third-party private or public insurers or from patients directly.

Staying financially nimble is important in a changing health care world. Progress in gaining efficiencies as well as effective service delivery is crucial to the future success of the ACO. Lawrence Casalino (2010), a noted health delivery system expert, has argued in a presentation at the New York Academy of Medicine, on April 15, 2010, that ACOs must not only be able to deliver services at reasonable cost but also have to continue to improve the quality of care. Therefore, to move in this direction, the third-party payers, mainly Medicare, have to be able to measure improvements and offer financial incentives to get ACOs to move in that direction. According to Casalino (2010, pp. 10–11), there are many unanswered questions about ACOs that need to be addressed by planners, including how patients will be assigned, how locked in they will be, how ACOs will be paid, what performance measures will be used, and what percentage of potential income will be at risk. In addition, the size of the ACO, its relationship with academic medical centers, whether provider market leverage will lead to increased costs, and can insurance plans participate are issues that need to be resolved. Finally, the relationship between ACOs and medical homes needs to be clearly articulated since people with chronic conditions are likely, given the evidence assembled in this book, to be better treated at the ACO if this model is adopted.

Casalino (2010, p. 19) further recommends that improvements in quality should be rewarded and ACOs should be tiered to promote risk taking in health care delivery at the service of the patient, which is a break from how ACOs will be supported by the Center for Medicare and Medicaid Services. What is being adapted to the ACO is the pay for performance model, with good health outcomes and evidence of care coordination being rewarded at large and moderate rates in a fully integrated delivery system. At the end of his presentation, Casalino warned the audience that tremendous organizational and cultural change is required as well as the need to incentivize to change specialist behavior and get hospitals on board the ACO express.

A few months later, Casalino joined Steven M. Shortell and Elliot S. Fisher, two other mandarins of health care payment and delivery reform, in an article laying out the options for accountable care organizations, given that the Center for Medicare and Medicaid Innovation will be seeking to create change in a health care system with uneven rates of development. (The language seems to be borrowed from the United States Treasury Department's "stress tests for banks.") Accountable care models constitute a continuum of risk, depending on the degree of organization found, so that integrated delivery system, which "involve a common ownership of hospitals, physician practices, and—in some cases—an insurance plan" (Shortell, Casalino, and Fisher, 2010, p. 1234) are more able to align financial incentives, electronic health records, team based care, and resources to support cost effective care, and therefore are in a better position to assume financial risk and seek rewards for doing so than small independent practitioners that may be linked only by a local medical foundation in rural areas. The authors also lay out other options that appear between the integrated delivery system and the linkage that might exist between small independent practitioners.

The idea of tiers is developed in this article as the authors posit that "the more-integrated forms of accountable care, such as integrated delivery systems and multispecialty group practices, are capable of assuming the greatest risk. This would make them natural candidates for capitation or bundled payments, in which providers assume a relatively greater share of risk" (Shortell, Casalino, and Fisher, 2010, p. 1295). Additionally, these organizations would also have the capacity and a large database to report on health outcomes and the impact of the services on the quality of life of patients.

Finally, the question of national affordability of continuing to allow ineffective procedures to continue will drive health policy, even if it is unstated. Health policy experts anticipate that the findings of the institute will be incorporated into the policies of public and private payers to attempt to eliminate the unsustainable rise in health care costs in the United States. It is anticipated that much will be done to remake the health care system so that it is not so disproportionately shaped by tertiary care and subspecialists, a recommendation that goes back to the 1970s to counterbalance the impact of Medicare on the U.S. health care system.

A great deal of health care reform is based on scaling up primary care through the patient-centered medical home. Yet there is no guarantee that primary care will become transformed in such as a way that all the incentives are aligned to benefit patients with chronic illnesses. Clearly, "major changes in the roles and relationships between primary care and the other components of the health care system" (Horner and Baron, 2010, p. 628) have to be brought about, outcomes that will take some time to establish.

The Affordable Care Act has also opened up the possibility that Medicare and Medicaid spending can be reduced while quality is maintained. It appears that the authors of the bill were listening to the health care delivery experts and made flexibility a built-in value during the implementation of the law.

> The HHS secretary is given the authority to expand the use of models like patient-centered medical homes within Medicare and Medicaid. She can do so if its been shown that these models reduce spending or the growth of spending without reducing quality, or can improve patient care without increasing spending. (Health Policy Brief , 2010b, p. 3)

Formal assessment or evaluation of projects will take place during the implementation of these demonstration projects. In the past, these new models were restricted financially so that federal expenditures were not to cost any more than prior service delivery efforts. Now demonstrations are not conducted under these limitations and the Center for Medicare and Medicaid Services is better funded to do the evaluations of medical homes as well as other innovations (Health Affairs, 2010, p. 4). And patient-centered medical homes are already being conceptualized as the foundation of the delivery system of the future within accountable care organizations.

The fingerprints of the health delivery system designers found on the ACA does not override the fingerprints of the health policy analysts. Not only is flexibility a characteristic of these ventures but participation with other funding streams is encouraged. The implementers at the CMS of the ACA hit the ground running in September 2010 by issuing solicitations for the Multi-payer Advanced Primary Care Initiative to locate states that will implement demonstration projects with which Medicare could be a partner (Health Affairs, 2010, p. 6).

Other health reform initiatives focus specifically on care coordination and seamless transitions from the hospital discharge to a return to one's home. There are grants available to hospitals with high admission rates to encourage them to form partnerships with community based medical groups. As identified by the AARP Public Policy Institute (2010),

> Grantees will be required to deliver at least one transitional care intervention, such as arranging post discharge services, providing patient self-management support (or caregiver support), or conducting medication management review. (p. 1)

The focus of these new services will be on high-risk beneficiaries in traditional fee-for-service Medicare.

Ending bad practices via penalties and rewards are also part of the provisions of the ACA. Medicare will also start in 2012 to create financial incentives by reducing payments to hospitals that cannot avoid unnecessary readmissions. A Medicare Independence at Home demonstration project will incentivize physicians and nurse practitioners to supply primary care services to patients at home. The financing of Medicaid health homes for chronic conditions is also part of the law, with these services including "care coordination, care management, transitional care and social support services, such as meals-on-wheels and Aging and Disability Resource Centers" (Lind, 2010, p. 3). An evaluation of this program will take place in 2017 to determine if there are reductions in emergency department visits, hospital admissions, and stays in skilled nursing homes, all ways of bending the cost curve. And independently of the third-party payers, interdisciplinary community health teams will be created to support medical homes, targeting patients with chronic conditions.

This is an ambitious agenda and the shift from fragmented to coordinated care is going to take years to complete. Much like trying to get a giant battleship or aircraft carrier turned around, changing the health care delivery system will not occur in a short time period. Improving chronic care will paradoxically require a reduction in expenditures and a smarter use of services so that we get better value for the money that is spent. This means eliminating unnecessary hospital admissions and avoiding preventable complications that are less likely to occur when the coordination of care and the use of information lead to a reduction of the number of bad decisions made by providers (Kocher and Sahni, 2010, p. 1).

The large integrated delivery systems required to make this efficient form of chronic care happen will be built on the foundations established in the ACA. Not only will more people be covered by 2014, but there will be initiatives established to drive a change in health care delivery, including patient-centered medical homes, accountable care organizations, bundled payments, readmissions reduction programs, and incentives to medical center managers to reduce hospital acquired conditions, all strong features of the ACA, as lucidly demonstrated by Kocher and Sahni (2010) in their table replicated as Table 10.1. There can be no progress toward universal coverage in the United States without movement to remake the health care system to accommodate the newly insured while offering improved care to all, especially people with chronic illnesses.

In sum, while some of the reforms in this comprehensive package of changes are transparently aimed at ending injustice and even the financial inequality that have increased in the United States during the past 30 years through creating health care security for more than 50 million Americans without health insurance, there is recognition in the Obama administration that we cannot continue uncontrolled spending, often the result of too much care, often coming from therapies that don't work or are only partially effective. Change is coming but the health care industry is large and powerful and often unwilling to accept change. The public also remains unconvinced by the prima

**Table 10.1**

| PERSPECTIVE: | PHYSICIANS VERSUS HOSPITALS AS LEADERS OF ACOs |
|---|---|

**By Robert Kocher and Nikhil R. Sahni**

### ACA Provisions Catalyzing a Shift from Fragmented Care to Coordinated Care

| Summary | Implications |
|---|---|
| **Patient-Centered Medical Homes (∫3502)** | |
| Community-based interdisciplinary, inter-professional teams that support primary care practices | Will drive improved organization of outpatient care |
| Government to provide grants or enter into contacts with eligible entities | Will fund care coordination and a team-based approach |
| **Accountable Care Organizations (∫3022)** | |
| Shared-savings program that encompasses primary care, specialist practice, and hospitals | Requires vertical coordination |
| Care processes to be redesigned for the efficient delivery of high-quality services | Most of the savings are likely to come from hospitals |
| **Bundled Payments (∫3023)** | |
| Pilot program | Will provide incentives for care-delivery systems to reduce costs in order to increase margins |
| Applicable to eight conditions selected by the secretary of health and human services | |
| An "episode of care" defined as the period from 3 days before admission through 30 days after discharge | |
| **Readmissions Reduction Program (∫3025)** | |
| Reduce payments for readmissions | Will motivate hospitals to engage with care coordinators and organize delivery systems better |
| Applicable to three conditions selected by the secretary of health and human services; to be expanded in 2015 | |
| Secretary to determine what is considered a readmission (i.e. minimum time between admissions) | |

*(continued)*

**Table 10.1    (Continued)**

| PERSPECTIVE: | PHYSICIANS VERSUS HOSPITALS AS LEADERS OF ACOs |
|---|---|
| **Hospital-Acquired Conditions (∫3008)** | |
| Payments for care for hospital-acquired conditions to be reduced, starting in 2015 | Will provide hospitals an incentive to standardize protocols and procedures to reduce hospital-acquired conditions |
| Individual hospitals' infection data to be made available online | |

*Source:* Reprinted from Physicians versus Hospitals as Leaders of Accountable Care Organizations, Robert Kocher and Nikhil R. Sahni, *New England Journal of Medicine*, November 12, 2010. Copyright © 2010 Massachusetts Medical Society.

facie merits of change, as evident in the Missouri referendum in July 2010 where voters rejected the Affordable Care Act. There need to be some facts on the ground for public opinion to warm to health care reform of this magnitude. The word has to be spread outside of the overly simplified, nonreality based, and often completely distorted statements about the ACA found in such venues as Fox News.

It is easy to sway large sectors of the public who only pay attention to politics during presidential elections, have given up reading newspapers, and fail to belong to voluntary associations, that is, organizations that have an interest in putting forth a coherent point of view about government and that can proffer an alternative view of reality. While the 2010 election was mostly about jobs, foreclosures, and resentment toward those who seemed to escape from hard times, there certainly are those who did find the Affordable Care Act another federal giveaway to the disinherited in our society. There were totally false claims and deliberate distortions courtesy of the members of the Tea Party and their media manipulators following the passage of the ACA that illegal immigrants would be covered by Medicaid expansion and that the state exchanges were going to issue them subsidized insurance policies. When the fear tactics prior to passage—death panels—didn't stop the development of the legislation, the Right turned to seeking to show that it was an income transfer to the undeserving low- and moderate-income uninsured, the first step to the spread of socialism in America. This immediate response to change shielded the portions of the ACA that seek to make for coordinated care, ending the dysfunctional structure of health care in America.

But not so fast, I have to say. There are laws on the books that were meant to protect the patients from doctors and hospitals who engage in price fixing, that try to hide poorly delivered care, or to permit fraudulent billing. Hospitals and independent practice associations that were feverishly creating ACOs in November and December 2010 sought to strike a balance by maintaining these older consumer protections and permitting organizational and clinical cooperation, forming new collectives, so that they can take advantage of the incentives found in the Affordable Care Act.

Vulnerable parts of the population are skeptical of the value of some of the proposed changes. Some disability advocates suggest that the newly formed ACOs will "cherry pick" and avoid the more expensive and difficult cases for bundled payments, even when there may be severe legal penalties established through the Center for Medicare and Medicaid Services that would discourage that kind of selectivity. There appears to be a new sheriff in town, or the country, CMS Director Dr. Donald M. Berwick who reassures the patient public that it will not happen. Still, the ACA is encouraging mergers, acquisitions, and partnerships between medical centers and doctors in the community that will keep many health law experts busy for the next decade (Pear, 2010).

Change leads to much exaggeration and fear, as we saw during the run-up to the passage of the ACA, especially during the summer of 2009. There is much to be done to convince the American people that limiting access to care that is proven to be effective is a good thing for them as patients, even if it may mean that they get less than was available for their parents; sometimes, less is more. Ineffective care can be dangerous to one's health. And as was also the case with the introduction of Medicare and Medicaid, the doubters came around to see the virtues of public options to address problems that the marketplace alone cannot solve.

# References

AARP Public Policy Institute (2010, November). Health reform initiatives to improve care coordination and transitional care for chronic conditions. Washington, D.C. Fact Sheet 191. AARP Public Policy Institute.

Abelson, R. (2009, May 9). Hospitals pay for cutting costly readmissions. *New York Times*, B1, B4.

Abelson, R. (2010a, October 20). Insurers test new cancer pay systems. *New York Times*, pp. B1, B8.

Abelson, R. (2010b, June 22). Paying to cut health costs: Extra nurses help doctors keep patients out of the hospital. *New York Times*, pp. B1, B7.

Adams, J. L., Mehrotra, A., Thomas, J. W., and McGlynn, E. A. (2010). Physician cost profiling—reliability and risk of misclassification. *New England Journal of Medicine*, 362, 1014–1021.

Adashi, E. Y., Geiger, H. J., and Fine, M. D. (2010, April 28). Health care reform and primary care—the growing importance of the community health center. *New England Journal of Medicine*, Retrieved from http://healthcarereform.nejm.org

Aiken, L. H. (2010, December 16). Nurses for the future. *New England Journal of Medicine*. Retrieved from http://nejm.org

Aizenman, N. C. (2010, August 6). Obama administration awards $159.1 million for training geriatric-care workers. *Washington Post*. Retrieved from http://www.washingtonpost.com

Albert Einstein College of Medicine. (2010). Einstein receives MacArthur Grant to study impact of housing on cardiovascular health. *Einstein News*. Retrieved from http://www.einsten.yu.edu/home/news

Alford, R. (1972, Winter). The political economy of health care: Dynamics without change. *Politics and Society*, 2, 1–38.

Alonzo-Zaldivar, R. (2009, October 29). Could "medical homes" bring order to health care? Associated Press. Retrieved from http://www.google.com/hostednews/ap/article/ALeqM5jeuQbQBHj_aFEIVBxtdlwEsNX

Anderson, G. (2005). Medicare and chronic conditions. *New England Journal of Medicine*, 353, 305–309.

Appleby, J. (2008, July 14). Old-fashioned docs inspire new "medical homes." *USA Today.* Retrieved from www.usatoday.com

Appleby, J. (2010, March 11). Insurers test plans that stress patient choices: Policies encourage treatments that do the most good. *USA Today*, pp. B1–B2.

Arvantes, J. (2010, July 29). Primary care initiatives helps save state Medicaid program millions. Illinois combines two programs to improve quality, save costs. *AAFP News Now.* Retrieved from http://www.aafp .org/online

Bachrach, D. (2009, July 8). National health reform through the lens of New York Medicaid. Paper presented at the United Hospital Fund Conference on Medicaid and National Health Reform, New York City.

Balogh, R., Hunter, D., and Quellette-Kuntz, H. (2005). Hospital utilization among persons with an intellectual disability, Ontario, Canada, 1995–2001. *Journal of Applied Research in Intellectual Disabilities*, 18, 181–190.

Barbour, A. B. (1995). *Caring for patients: A critique of the medical model.* Stanford, CA: Stanford University Press.

Baron, R. J. (2009). The chasm between intention and achievement in primary care. *Journal of the American Medical Association*, 301, 1922–1924.

Baron, R. J., and Cassel, C. K. (2008). 21st century primary care: New physician roles need new payment models. *Journal of the American Medical Association*, 299, 1595–1597.

Barry, P. (2009). The new face of health care. *AARP Bulletin* (April), 12–14.

Berenson, A. (2010a, February 10). The world of long-term care hospitals. Facilities proliferate across U.S. but without much scrutiny. *New York Times*, pp. A1, A13, A14.

Berenson, A. (2010b, February 10). Trail of disquieting reports from hospitals of Select Medical. *New York Times*, p. A14.

Berenson, R. (2006). *Challenging the status quo in chronic disease care: Seven case studies.* Oakland, CA: California HealthCare Foundation.

Berenson, R., and Howell, J. (2009, July). Structuring, financing and paying for effective chronic care coordination. Executive Summary. A Report Commissioned by the National Coalition on Care Coordination (N3C0). Washington, DC: National Coalition on Care Coordination.

Berenson, R. A., and Rich, E. C. (2010). US approaches to physician payment: The deconstruction of primary care. *Journal of General Internal Medicine*, 25, 613–618.

Berk, M. L., and Monheit, A. C. (2001). The concentration of health care expenditures, revisited. *Health Affairs*, 20, 9–18.

Bernstein, J., Chollet, D., Peikes, D., and Peterson, G. G. (2010, June). *Medical homes: Will they improve primary care? Issue brief.* Princeton, NJ: Mathematica Policy Research.

Berwick, D. M. (2009, May 19). What "patient-centered" should mean: Confessions of an extremist. *Health Affairs web exclusive*, pp. W555–563. Retrieved from http://www.HealthAffairswebexclusive

Bindman, A. B., Chattopadhyay, A., and Auerback, G. M. (2008). Interruptions in Medicaid coverage increase and risk of hospitalization. *Annals of Internal Medicine*, 149, 854–860.

Birenbaum, A. (1990). *In the shadow of medicine. Remaking the division of labor in health care*. Dix Hills, NY: General Hall.

Birenbaum, A. (2002). *Wounded profession: American medicine enters the age of managed care*. Westport, CT: Praeger.

Bitsko, R. H., Visser, S. N., Schieve, L. A., Ross, D. S., Thurman, D. J., and Perou, R. (2009). Unmet health care needs among CSHCN with neurologic conditions. *Pediatrics Supplement*, 4, 124, S343–351.

Bitton, A., Martin, C., and Landon, B. E. (2010). A nationwide survey of patient centered medical home demonstration projects. *Journal of General Internal Medicine*, 25, 584–592.

Blueprint. (2009, Spring). Next step in care: Involving families, improving quality. New York: United Hospital Fund, pp. 1–2.

Bodenheimer, T., and Berry-Millet, R. (2009). *Care management of patients with complex health care needs*. The Synthesis Project. New Insights from Research Results. Princeton, NJ: Robert Wood Johnson Foundation.

Bodenheimer, T., Wagner, E., and Grumbach, K. (2002a). Improving primary care for patient with chronic illness. *Journal of the American Medical Association*, 288, 1775–1779.

Bodenheimer, T., Wagner, E., and Grumbach, K. (2002b). Improving primary care for patients with chronic illness: The chronic care model, part 2. *Journal of the American Medical Association*, 228, 1909–1914.

Bodenheimer, T., and West, D. (2010, October 7). Low-cost lessons from Grand Junction, Colorado. *New England Journal of Medicine*, 363, 1391–1393.

Bohmer, R. M. J., and Lee, T. H. (2009). The shifting mission of health care delivery organizations. *New England Journal of Medicine*, 359, 1347–1349.

Boult, C., and Wieland, G. D. (2010). Comprehensive primary care for older patients with multiple chronic conditions. *Journal of the American Medical Association*, 304, 1936–1943.

Boutwell, A. (2010, April 1). Letter to the editor on discharge planning and rates of readmissions. *New England Journal of Medicine*, 362, 1244.

Brody, J. E. (2010, February 23). Medical paper trail takes electronic turn. *New York Times*, p. D7.

Brook, R. H. (2009). The science of health care reform. *Journal of the American Medical Association*, 301, 2486–2487.

Buckley. L. M. (2008). *Talking with patients about the personal impact of illness: The doctor's role*. New York: Radcliffe Publishing.

California Health Care Foundation Almanac Update. (2010, July). California Physician Facts and Figures. Retrieved from www.chcf.org

Campbell, C. A. (2009, March 9). An ER alternative. Retrieved from Philly.com, pp. 1–4.

Casale, A., Paulus, R. A., Selna, M. J., Doll, M. C., Bothe, A. E., Jr., McKinley, K. E., Berry, S. A., Davis, E. E., Gilfillan, R. J., Hamory, B. H., and Steele, G. D., Jr. (2007 October). ProvenCare SM: A provider-driven pay for performance program for acute episodic cardiac surgical care. *Annals of Surgery*, 246, 613–623.

Casalino, L. P. (2010, April 15). Accountable care organizations: Models and issues. A slide presentation at a panel on accountable care organizations at the New York Academy of Medicine. New York City. Slides made available courtesy of Dr. Casalino.

Cassel, C. K. (2009). Policy for an aging society. *Journal of the American Medical Association*, 302, 2701–2702.

Chase, D. (2010a). Montefiore Medical Center: Integrated care delivery for vulnerable populations. Case Study of the Integrated Safety-Net Health Care System. The Commonwealth Fund (October), New York.

Chase, D. (2010b, December 22). *Patients gain information and skills to improve self-management through innovative tools. Quality matters.* New York: Commonwealth Fund. Retrieved from http://www.commonwealthfund.org/Content/Newsletters/Quality-Matters/2010/December

Chen, P. W. (2010, July 15). Putting patients at the center of the medical home. Retrieved from http://www.nytimes.com/2010/07/15/health/15chen.html?

Ciechanowksi, P. S., Katon, W. J., and Russo, J. E. (2000). Depression and diabetes: Impact of depression symptoms on adherence, function, and costs. *Archives of Internal Medicine*, 160, 3278–3285.

Cleland, J. G. F., and Ekman, I. (2010). Enlisting the help of the largest health care workforce—patients. *Journal of the American Medical Association*, 304, 1383–1384.

Committee on the Future Health Care Workforce for Older Americans. (2008). *Retooling for an aging America: Building the health care workforce.* Washington, DC: National Academies Press.

Commonwealth Fund. (2010, June 24). Case study: The Mount Auburn Cambridge Independent Practice Association. Retrieved from www.commonwealthfund.org/Content/Newsletters/Quality-Matters/2010June/July

Commonwealth Fund Commission on a High Performance Health System. (2009, November 20). Keeping both eyes on the prize: Expanding coverage and changing the way we pay for care are essential to make health reform work for families and businesses. Retrieved from www.commonwealthfund.org/Content/Publications/Other/2009/Keeping-Both-Eye

Consortium for Citizens with Disabilities Health Task Force. (2010, August 26). Draft of an unpublished letter to the Office of Consumer Information and Oversight, Department of Health and Human Services, pp. 1–4.

Costello, D. J., Girion, L., and Hiltzik, M. A. (2008, October 23). The battle of the medical bills. *Los Angeles Times*. Retrieved from www.latimes.com

Cromwell, J., et al. (1998). Medicare participating health bypass demonstration: Final report. Baltimore, MD: Center on Medicare and Medicaid Services.

Cubanski, J., and Neuman, P. (2010, August 12). Medicare doesn't work as well for younger, disabled beneficiaries as it does for older enrollees. Retrieved from http://healthaffairs.org/cgi/content/full/hlthaff.2009.0962vl

Cunningham, P. J. (2009, July). Chronic burdens: The persistently high out-of-pocket health care expenses faced by many Americans with chronic conditions. Issue Brief. New York. Commonwealth Fund, 63, 1–13.

Cunningham, P. J. (2010a). Explaining the increase in family financial pressures from medical bills between 2003 and 2007: Do affordability thresholds change over time? *Medical Research and Review, 20*, 1–15.

Cunningham, P. J. (2010b). The growing financial burden of health care: National and state trends, 2001–2006. *Health Affairs, 29*, 1037–1044.

Cylus, J., Hartman, M., Washington, B., Andrews, K., and Catlin, A. (2010, December). Pronounced gender and age differences are evident in personal health care spending per person. *Health Affairs, 30*, 153–160.

Dall, T. M., Zhang, Y., Chen, Y. J., Quick, W. W., Yang, W. G., and Fogli, J. (2010). Chronic disease. The economic burden of diabetes. *Health Affairs, 29*, 297–303.

Dartmouth Atlas of Health Care. (2006). *Variation among states in the management of severe chronic illness.* Hanover, NH: Author, Dartmouth College.

Davis, K. (2010, August 2). Coherent and transparent health care payment: Sending the right signals in the marketplace. *The Commonwealth Fund Blog.* Retrieved from http://www.commonwealthfund-All.aspx?author=Davis+Karen

Davis, K., and Collins, S. (2010, March 22). A new era in American health care. Retrieved from The Commonwealth Fund Blog.

Davis, K, Schoen, C., and Stemikis, K. (2010, June). *Mirror, mirror on the wall: How the performance of the U.S. health care system compares internationally.* 2010 Update. New York: Commonwealth Fund.

deBrantes, F., Rosenthal, M. B., and Painter, M. (2009). Perspectives: Building a bridge from fragmentation to accountability—the Prometheus payment model. *New England Journal of Medicine, 361*, 1033–1036.

DeGuire, P., Lee, C., Rafferty, A. P., and Fussman, C. (2008). Health status of Michigan adults with disabilities. *Michigan BFRSS Surveillance Brief. 2.* Lansing, MI: Michigan: Department of Community Health, Chronic Disease Epidemiology Section.

Dentzer, S. (2010a). Reinventing primary care: A task that is far "too important to fail." *Health Affairs, 29*, 757–759.

Dentzer, S. (2010b). The California HealthCare Foundation pursues a broad agenda. *Health Affairs, 29*, 291–296.

Dentzer, S. (2010c). Geisinger chief Glenn Steele seizing health reform's potential to build a superior system. *Health Affairs, 29*, 1200–1207.

Dentzer, S. (2010d). An international focus and a retrospective on change. *Health Affairs, 29*, 2136–2137.

DeVol, R., and Bedroussian, A. (2007). *An unhealthy America: The economic burden of chronic disease: Charting a new course to save the lives and increase productivity and economic growth.* N.p.: The Milken Institute.

Dreifus, C. (2010, November 30). A nephrologist and patient. *New York Times,* p. D2.

Dunn, H. R. (2010). Health behavior vs. the stress of low socioeconomic status and health outcomes. *Journal of the American Medical Association, 303*, 1199–1200.

Ehlenbach, W. J., Hough, C. L., Crane, P. K., Haneuse, S., Carson, S. C., Curtis, J. R., and Larson, E. B. (2010). Association between acute care and critical hospitalization and cognitive function in older adults. *Journal of the American Medical Association*, 303, 763–770.

Emerson, E. (2009). Relative child poverty, income inequality, wealth, and health. *Journal of the American Medical Association*, 301, 425–426.

Epstein, A. M. (2009). Revisiting readmissions—changing the incentives for shared accountability. *New England Journal of Medicine*, 360, 1457–1459.

Epstein, R. M., Fiscella, K., Lesser, C. S., and Stange, K. C. (2010). Analysis and commentary: Why the nation needs a policy push on patient-centered health care. *Health Affairs*, 29, 1489–1495.

Fairman, J. A., Rowe, J. W., Hassmiller, S., and Shalala, D. E. (2010, December 16). Broadening the scope of nursing practice. *New England Journal of Medicine*. Retrieved from www.nejm.org, pp. 1–4

Ferrie, J. E., Martikainen, P., Shipley, M. J., Marmot, M. G., Stansfeld, S. A., and Smith G. D. (2001). Employment status and health after privatization in white collar civil servants: Prospective cohort study. *British Medical Journal*, 322, 647–651.

Fisher, E. S., and Shortell, S. M. (2010). Accountable care organizations: Accountable for what, to whom, and how. *Journal of the American Medical Association*, 304, 1715–1716.

Foubister, V. (2010, February). In focus: Health care institutions are slowly learning to listen to customers. The Commonwealth Fund Newsletter, pp. 1–4.

Fox, S., and Purcell, K. (2010, March 24). Chronic disease and the Internet. Pew Internet. Retrieved from http://pew internet.org

Freeman, S. (2010, October 14). A new theory of justice. *New York Review of Books*, 58, 58–60.

Freudenheim, M. (2009, December 22). Tool in cystic fibrosis fight: A registry. *New York Times*, pp. D1, D6.

Freudenheim, M. (2010, June 29). Preparing more care for an aging population. *New York Times*, pp. D5–6.

Friedberg, M. W., Coltin, K. L., Safran, D. G., Dresser, M., and Schneider, E. C. (2010). Medical home capabilities of primary care practices that serve sociodemographically vulnerable neighborhoods. *Archives of Internal Medicine*, 170, 938–944.

Friedberg, M. W., Hussey, P. S., and Schneider, E. C. (2010). Primary care: A critical review of the evidence on quality and cost of health care. *Health Affairs*, 29, 766–772.

Fuchs, V. R. (2008). Three "inconvenient truths" about health care. *New England Journal of Medicine*, 359, 1749–1751.

Gabel, J., Whitmore, H., and Pickreign, J. (2010, November). *Decade of decline: A survey of employer health insurance coverage in New York State*. New York: New York State Health Care Foundation, pp. 1–60.

Galobardes, B., Lunch, J. W., and Davey Smith, G. (2008). Is the association between childhood socioeconomic circumstance and cause-specific mortality established? An update of a systematic review. *Journal of Epidemiology and Community Health*, 62, 387–390.

Ganguli, I. (2010). The case for primary care—a medical student's perspective. *New England Journal of Medicine*, 363, 207–209.

Gardner, H. (2008, October 16). Infant deaths drop in U.S., but rate is still high. *New York Times*. Retrieved from http://www.nytimes.com/208/10/16/health/16infant.html

Gawande, A. (2009, December 14). Dept of Medicine. Testing, Testing. The health-care bill has no master plan for curbing costs. Is that a bad thing? *New Yorker*, pp. 34–40.

Gawande, A. (2010, August 2). Letting go: What should medicine do when it can't save your life? *New Yorker*, pp. 36–49.

Georgetown University Health Policy Institute. (2009). How the FEHBP Blue Cross Blue Shield Standard Option Plan covers medical care for patients with serious chronic conditions. Washington, DC: American Cancer Society Cancer Action Network.

Glazier, W. (1973, April). The task of medicine. *Scientific American*, 13–17.

Gold, J., and Galewitz, P. (2010a). Health care providers, insurers: Accountable care organizations bring legal worries. *Kaiser Health News*. Retrieved from http://www.kaiserhealthnews.org/Stories/2010/October/05/accountable care-organizations

Gold, J., and Galewitz, P. (2010b). Health care interests push to make ACOs pay off for them. *Kaiser Health News*. Retrieved from http://www.kaiserhealthnews.org/Stories/2010/October/11/health-care-interests

Goldsmith, J. (2010). Analyzing shifts in economic risks to providers in proposed payment and delivery system reforms. *Health Affairs*, 29, 7, 1299–1304.

Grady, D. (2010, August 4). Obesity rates keep rising, troubling health officials. *New York Times*, p. A11.

Greenlee, M. C. (2010, October 21). *The PCHM-neighbor: The interface of PCMH with specialty/subspecialty practices.* A paper presented at the Patient-Centered Primary Care Conference, Washington, DC.

Grumbach, K., and Grundy, P. (2010). *Outcomes of implementing patient centered medical home interventions: A review of the evidence from prospective evaluation studies in the United States.* (Updated, November 16). Washington, DC: Patient-Centered Primary Care Collaborative, pp. 1–16.

Ha, T., Boukus, E. R., and Cohen, G. (2010, December). Workplace clinics: A sign of growth employer interest in wellness. Research Brief Number 17. Washington, DC: Center for Studying Health System Change.

Hackbarth, G., Reischauer, R., and Mutti, A. (2008). Collective accountability for medical care—toward bundled Medicare payments. *New England Journal of Medicine*, 359, 3–5.

Halfon, N., and Newacheck, P.W. (2010). Evolving notions of childhood chronic illness. *Journal of the American Medical Association*, 303, 665–666.

Harris, G. (2008). Infant deaths drop in U.S. but rate is still high. *New York Times*. Retrieved from nytimes.com/2008/10/16/health/16infant.html?, 1–2

Hartzband, P., and Groopman, J. (2009). Keeping the patient in the equation—Humanism and health care reform. *New England Journal of Medicine*, 361, 554–555.

Hayes, E. (2010). Pre-existing condition insurance plan: HealthBridge NY. Health Bureau. New York State Insurance Department. Paper presented at the monthly meeting of New Yorkers for Affordable Health Care Meeting, July 20, 2010. New York City.

Health Policy Brief. (2010a, October 5). Comparative effectiveness research: A broad effort is under way to understand what really works in health care, perhaps leading to better value for dollar spent. HealthAffairs.org. Retrieved from www.HealthAffairs.org

Health Policy Brief. (2010b, September 14). Health policy brief: Patient centered medical homes. A new way to deliver primary care may be more affordable and improve quality. But how widely adopted will the model be? Retrieved from http://www.healthaffairs.org/healthpolicybriefs

Health Resources and Services Administration. (2009). The National Survey of Children with Special Health Care Needs Chartbook, 2005–2006. Silver Springs, MD: Maternal and Child Health Bureau, HRSA.

Health Resources and Services Administration. (2010). National Survey of Children with Special Health Care Needs 2005–2006. Retrieved from http://mchb.hrsa.gov

Hilderbrant, C. (2009, June 27). Health care services delivered at home can save on costs. Retrieved from DemocratandChronicle.com

Hof, P. R., Bouras, C., Perl, D. P., Sparks, I., Mehta, N., and Morrison, H. (1995). Age related distribution of neuropathologic changes on the cerebral cortex of patients with Down's syndrome. *Archives of Neurology*, 52, 379–391.

Hoffman, A., and Pearson, S. D. (2009, June 23). "Marginal medicine": Targeting comparative effectiveness research to reduce waste. *Health Affairs*, Web exclusive, w710–w718. Retrieved from www.HealthAffairs.org

Hollingsworth, B. (2010, March 1). Medicaid cuts strike a blow—Slashes in reimbursement for wheelchairs. Retrieved from the *Topeka Capital-Journal* through findarticles.com

Holsopple, K. (2010). *The Vermont Family Support 360 Project*. Waterbury, VT: Vermont Agency of Human Services, State of Vermont, pp. 1–2.

Holt, J., Esquivel, M., and Pariseau, C. (2010, July 12). *Medical Home Competencies for LEND Trainees*. Draft of an unpublished working paper. Salt Lake City, UT: Utah LEND Program, University of Utah.

Homer, C. J., and Baron, R. J. (2010). How to scale up primary care transformation: What we know and what we need to know. *Journal of General Internal Medicine*, 25, 625–629.

Homer, C. J., Kaltka, K., Romm, D., Kuhlthau, Bloom, S., Newacheck, P., Van Cleave, J., and Perrin, J. M. (2008). A review of the evidence for the medical home for children with special health care needs. *Pediatrics*, 122, e922–e937. Retrieved from www.pediatrics.org

Iglehart, J. K. (2008). Medicare, graduate medical education, and new policy directions. *New England Journal of Medicine*, 359, 643–650.

Iglehart, J. K. (2010a, July 21). Health reform, primary care, and graduate medical education. *New England Journal of Medicine*. Retrieved from http://www.healthcarereform.nejm.org

Iglehart, J. K. (2010b). Perspective: Assessing an ACO prototype—Medicare's Physician Group Practice demonstration. *New England Journal of Medicine*, 362. Retrieved from http://healthpolicyandreform.nejm.org/?p=13455 &query=home

Issacs, S. L., and Schroeder, S. A. ( 2004). Class—the ignored determinant of the nation's health. *New England Journal of Medicine*, 351, 1137–1142.

Jauhar, S. (2009, December 1). To curb repeat hospital stays, pay doctors. *New York Times*, p. D6.

Jiang, W., Krishnan, R. R., and O'Connor, C. M. (2002). Depression and heart disease: Evidence of a link and its therapeutic implication. *CNS Drugs*, 16, 111–127.

Kaiser Family Foundation. (2009, October 21). News Release. Growing numbers of Americans report problems paying medical bills and delaying and skipping care due to costs. Washington, DC: Kaiser Family Foundation. Retrieved from kff.org

Kaiser Health News Staff. (2010, March 31). True or false: Seven concerns about the new health law. Retrieved from KaiserHealthNews.org

Kanaan, S. B. (2008). Promoting effective self-management approaches to improve chronic disease care: Lessons learned. Oakland, CA: California HealthCare Foundation.

Kindig, D. A., Asada, Y., and Booske, B. (2008). A population health framework for setting national and state goals. *Journal of the American Medical Association*, 299, 17, 2081–2083.

Klein, S. (2010, June 24). In focus: Building accountable care organizations that improve quality and lower costs—a view from the field. Retrieved from www.commonwealthfund.org/Quality-Matters/2010/June and July

Kocher, R., and Sahni, N. R. (2010, November 12). Perspective: Physicians versus hospitals as leaders of accountable care organizations. Retrieved from www.nejm.org

Kogan, M. D., Newacheck, P. W., Blumberg, S. J., Ghandour, R. M., Singh, G. K., Strckland, B. B., and van Dyck, P. C. (2010, August 26). Underinsurance among children in the United States. *New England Journal of Medicine*, 363, 841–851.

Kogan, M. D., Strickland, B. B., and Newacheck, P. W. (2009). Building systems of care: Findings from the national survey of children with special health care needs. *Pediatrics Supplement*, 4, 124, S333–S336.

Konrad, W. (2010, July 24). For chronic care, try turning to your employer. *New York Times*, p. B6.

Krisky-McHale, S. J., Devenny, D. A., Gu, H, Jenkins, E. C., Murty, V. V., Schupf, N., Scotto, L., Tycko, B., Urv, T. K., Ye, L., Zigman, W. B., and Silverman, W. (2008). Successful aging in a 70-year-old man with Down Syndrome: A case study. *Intellectual and Developmental Disabilities*, 46, 215–228.

Landefeld, C. S., Winker, M. A., and Chernof, B. (2009). Clinical care in the aging century—announcing care of the gaining patient: From evidence to action. *Journal of the American Medical Association*, 302, 2703–2704.

Landers, S. H. (2010, October 21). Perspective: Why health care is going home. *New England Journal of Medicine.* Retrieved from http://www.nejm.org/doi/ful/10.1056/NEJMp100401

Landrigan, C. P., Parry, G. J., Bones, C. B., Hackbarth, A. D., Goldmann, D. A., and Sharek, P. J. (2010). Temporal trends in rates of patient harm resulting from medical care. *New England Journal of Medicine, 363,* 2124–2134.

Laraque, D., and Sia, C. J. (2010). Health care reform and the opportunity to implement a family-centered medical home for children. *Journal of the American Medical Association, 303,* 2407–2408.

Larson, E. B., and Reid, R. (2010). The patient centered medical home movement: Why now? *Journal of the American Medical Association, 303,* 1644–1645.

Lee, P. V., Berenson, R. A., and Tooker, J. (2009). Payment reform—the need to harmonize approaches in Medicare and the private sector. Posted by the *New England Journal of Medicine.* Retrieved from http://healthcarereform.nejm.org

Leon, K., McDonald, L. K., Moore, B., and Rust, G. (2009). Disparities in influenza treatment among disabled Medicaid patients in Georgia. *American Journal of Public Health, Supplement 2, 99,* S378–382.

Leonhardt, D. (2009, November 8). Dr. James will make it better. *New York Times Magazine,* pp. 31–37, pp. 44–47.

Leonhardt, D. (2010a, April 6). In medicine, the power of no. *New York Times,* p. B1.

Leonhardt, D. (2010b, October 20). Proving innovation in Medicare. *New York Times,* pp. B1, B8.

Levine, J. M. (2009, July 8). *Challenges to integrating behavioral health and primary care. Presented at the United Hospital Fund Symposium.* Paper presented at the conference on Medicaid and National Health Reform. New York City.

Lewin Group. (2010, July). Bending the health care cost curve in New York State: Options for saving money and improving care. New York: NYS Health Foundation.

Lewis, M. (2009, July 24) Is becoming a medical home worth the trouble? Medical homes can mean more money, but they're not for everyone. *Medical Economics,* pp. 1–6.

Lind, K. D. (2010, May). Health reform initiatives to improve care coordination and transitional care for chronic conditions. Fact Sheet 191. Washington, DC: American Association of Retired People's Public Policy Institute.

Long, K. R., Ritter, P. Stewart, A. L., Sobel, D. S., Brown, B. W., Bandura, A. Gonzalez, V. M., Laurent, D. D., and Holman, H. R. (2001). Chronic disease self-management program: 2-year health status and health care utilization outcomes. *Medical Care, 39,* 1217–1223.

Lorig, K. R., Sobel, D. S., Steward, A. L., Brown, B. W., Jr., Bandura, A, Ritter, P. Gonzalez, V. M., Laurent D. D., and Holman, H. R. (1999). Evidence suggesting that a chronic disease self-management program can improve health status while reducing hospitalization: A randomized trial. *Journal of Medical Care, 37,* 5–14.

Lubkin, I. M., and Larsen, P. D. (2006). *Chronic illness: Impact and interventions.* Sixth edition. Sudbury, MA: Jones and Bartlett Publishers.

Luft, H. S. (2009). Health care reform—toward more freedom and responsibility for physicians. *New England Journal of Medicine*, 361, 623–628.

Lui, C., and Wallace, S. P. (2010, March). Chronic conditions of Californians. 2007 California Health Interview Survey. Oakland, CA: California HealthCare Foundation.

Macinko, J., Dourado, I., Auino, R., de Fatima Bonolo, P., Lima-Costa, M. F., Medina, G. M., Mota, E., Berenice de Oliveira, V., and Turci, M. A. (2010). Major expansion of primary care in Brazil linked to decline in unnecessary hospitalization. *Health Affairs*, 29, 2149–2160.

Mackenbach, J. P., Stirbu, I., and Roskam, A-JR, Schaap, M. M., Menvielle, W., Leinsalu, M., and Kunst, A. E. (2008). Socioeconomic inequalities in health in 22 European countries. *New England Journal of Medicine*, 358, 2468–2481.

Mandl, K. D., and Kohane, I. S. (2008). Techtonic shifts in the health information economy. *New England Journal of Medicine*, 358, 1730–1737.

Mann, J. J. (2005). Drug therapy: The medical management of depression. *New England Journal of Medicine*, 353, 1810–1834.

Marcus, A. D. (2004a, September 8). New approaches to lung cancer: Being aggressive. *The Wall Street Journal*, p. A1.

Marcus, A. D. (2004b, June 9). Next chapter. After leukemia, family struggles to define "normal." *The Wall Street Journal*, p. A1.

Marcus, A. D. (2004c, September 8). Science and health. A wife's struggle with cancer takes an unexpected toll. *The Wall Street Journal*, p. A1.

Marmot, M. (2005). Social determinants of health. *The Lancet*, 365, 1099–1104.

McLaughlin, T. (2010, December 14). Personal communication via e-mail.

Medicare Rights Center. (2010). Getting Medicare right: Side-by-side comparison of health reform bills' impact on Medicare. Washington, DC: Medicare Rights Center.

Merlis, M. (2010, July 27). Health policy brief: Accountable care organizations. Under the health reform law, Medicare will be able to contract with these to provide care to enrollees. What are they and how will they work? Accessed from www.healthaffairs.org

Merrell, K., and Berenson, R. A. (2010). Structuring payments for medical homes. *Health Affairs*, 29, 852–858.

Meyer, H. (2010). Report from the field. Group Health's move to the medical home: For doctors, it's often a hard journey. *Health Affairs*, 29, 844–851.

Miller, C. C. (2010, March 24). Social networks: A lifeline for the chronically ill. *New York Times*. Retrieved from http://www.nytimes.com

Minot, J. (2009, October). Policy brief: Geographic variation and health care cost growth: Research to inform a complex diagnosis. *Changes in Health Care Financing and Organization*, Princeton, NJ: Robert Wood Johnson Foundation.

Mitchell, E. (2009, October 28). *Getting what we pay for: Moving to value based payment in Maine.* Paper presented at the New York State Health Care Foundation Conference.

M M Link. Personal Approaches to Primary Care. Well Blog. New York Times .com. Retrieved from http://well.blogs.nytimes.com/2010/07/15/ a-personal-approach-to-primary-care/

Mor, V., Intrator, O., Feng, Z., and Grabowski, D. C. (2010). The revolving door of rehospitalization from skilled nursing facilities. *Health Affairs*, 29, 57–64.

Moster, D., Lie, R. T., and Markestad, T. (2008). Long-term medical and social consequences of preterm birth. *New England Journal of Medicine*, 359, 262–273.

Naylor, M. D., Brooten, D. A., Campbell, R. L., Maislin, G., McCauley, K. M., and Schwartz, J. S. (2004). Transitional care of older adults hospitalized with heart failure: A randomized, control trial. *Journal of the American Geriatric Society*, 52, 675–684.

Neumann, P. J., and Tunis, S. R. (2010). Medicare and medical technology— the growing demand for relevant outcomes. *New England Journal of Medicine*, 362, 377–379.

New York Times. (2009, December 30). Editorial: The case for reform. *The New York Times*, p. A26.

New York Times. (2010a, December 12). Editorial: Health care and the deficit. *New York Times*, p. wk 7.

New York Times. (2010b, July 15). A personal approach to primary care. Retrieved from http://well.blogs.nytimes.com/2010/07/15/a-personal -approach-to-primary-care/

NYS Health Foundation. (2010, October, 5). Bending the cost curve in New York State: Implementation plan to adopt bundled payment methods. NYS Health Foundation. Retrieved from http://www.NYS HealthFoundation.org

Orszag, P. (2010, December 10). Making disability work. *New York Times*, p. A35.

Paeglow, T. (2007). School of Public Health, University at Albany State University of New York. Disability and Health: Implications for Public Health Practice. Retrieved from www.t2b2.org

Paez, K. A., Zhao, L., and Hwang, W. (2009). Rising out-of-pocket spending for chronic conditions: A ten-year trend. *Health Affairs*, 28, 26–35.

Parekh, A. K., and Barton, M. (2010). The challenge of multiple comorbidity for the US health care system. *Journal of the American Medical Association*, 303, 1303–1304.

Parish, S. L., Rose, R. A., Grinstein-Weiss, M., and Andrews, M. E. (2008). Material hardship in U.S. families raising children with disabilities. *Exceptional Children*, 75, 71–92.

Patient-Centered Primary Care Collaborative. (2007). Joint Principles of the Patient Centered Medical Home. Retrieved from http://pcpcc.net

Patient-Centered Primary Care Collaborative. (2009, February 24). Pennsylvania Chronic Care Initiative. Retrieved from http://www.pcpcc.net

Patient Protection and Affordable Care Act. HR3590. 2010.

Paulus, R. A., Davis, K., and Steele, G. D.(2008). Continuous innovation in health care: Implications of the Geisinger experience. *Health Affairs*, 27, 1235–1246.

Pear, R. (2010, November 20). Consumer risks feared as health law spurs mergers. *New York Times*, p. A18.

Perspectives. (2008). The future of primary care—the community responds. *New England Journal of Medicine*, 359, 2636–2638.

Pham, H. H., Schrag, D., O'Malley, A. S., Wu, B., and Bach, P. B. (2007). Care patterns in Medicare and their implications for pay for performance. *New England Journal of Medicine*, 356, 1130–1139.

Pignone, M. P., Gaynes B. N., Rushton J. L., Burchell C. M., Orleans C. T., Mulrow, C. D., and Lohr, K. N. (2002). Screening for depression in adults: A summary of the evidence from the U.S. Preventive Services Task Force. *Annals of Internal Medicine*, 136, 765–776.

Powell, L. H., Calvin, J. E., Jr., Richardson, D., Janssen, I., Mendes de Leon, C. F., Flynn, K. J., Grady, K. L., Rucker-Whitaker, C. S., L. K., Eaton, C., and Avery, E. (2010). Self-management counseling in patients with heart failure. The heart failure adherence and retention randomized behavioral trial. *Journal of the American Medical Association*, 304, 1331–1338.

Pulse. (2010, April). Association of Maternal and Child Health Programs. Washington, DC: Author, p. 11.

Rabin, R. C. (2010a, June 8). Enlisting patients in the fight to cut costs. *New York Times*, p. E4.

Rabin, R. C. (2010b, May 18). In health law, a clearer view of coverage. *New York Times*, p. D6.

Ramer, H. (2010, July 15). NH to test health care collaboration at 5 sites. Bloomberg Businessweek. Retrieved from www.businessweek

Rau, J. (2008, August 4). Health ambition narrows. *Los Angeles Times*. Retrieved from www.latimes.com

Raven, M. (2009, October, 28). *Improving care and cutting costs for high-risk Medicaid patients*. Paper presented at the New York State Health Care Foundation Conference, New York City.

Reichard, J. (2010a, July 15). Health care law's accountable care groups attract rare bipartisan flavor. *Congressional Quarterly*. Retrieved from www .commonwealthfund.org/Content/Newsletters/Washington-Health -Policy-in-Review

Reichard, J. (2010b, May 24). Hospital alliance kicks off big test of health delivery redesign. Retrieved from http://www.commonwealthfund.org

Reichard, J. (2010c, September 13). Primary care access doesn't by itself equal better treatment, Dartmouth study says. Retrieved from http://www .commonwealthfund.org/Content/Newsletters/Washington-Health -Policy-in-Review

Reid, R. J., Coleman, K., Johnson, E. A., Fishman, P. A., Hsu, C., Soman, M. P., Trescott, C. E., Erikson, M., and Larson, E. B. (2010). The Group Health medical home at year two: Cost savings, higher patient satisfaction, and less burnout for providers. *Health Affairs*, 29, 835–843.

Reid, R. J., Fishman, P. A., Onchee, Y., Ross, T. R., Tufano, J. T., Soman, M. P., and Larson, E. B. (2009). Patient-centered medical home demonstration: A prospective, quasi-experimental, before and after evaluation. *American Journal of Managed Care*, 15, e71–e87.

Reid, T. R. (2009). *The healing of America: A global quest for better, cheaper, and fairer health care*. New York: Penguin Press.

Reuben, D. B. (2009). Medical care for the final years of life. "When you're 83, its not going to be 20 years." *Journal of the American Medical Association*, 302, 2686–2694.

Rittenhouse, D. R., Casalino, L. P., Gilles, R. R., Shortell, S. M., and Lau, B. (2008). Measuring the medical home infrastructure in large medical groups. *Health Affairs*, 27, 1246–1258.

Rittenhouse, D. R., Shortell, S. M., and Fisher, E. S. (2009). Primary care and accountable care—Two essential elements of delivery-system reform. *New England Journal of Medicine*. Retrieved from http://healthreform.nejm.org

Rittenhouse, D. R., Thorn, D. H., and Schmittdiel, J. A. (2010). Developing a policy-relevant research agenda for the patient centered medical home: A focus on outcomes. *Journal of General Internal Medicine*, 25, 593–600.

Robert Wood Johnson Foundation (2010, November). Health care consumer confidence index. Princeton, NJ: Author, pp. 1–18.

Rosland, A. M. (2009). Sharing the care: The role of the family in chronic illness. Oakland, CA: California Health Care Foundation.

Rosser, W. W., Cowill, J. M., Kasperski, J., and Wilson, L. (2010). Patient-centered medical homes in Ontario. *New England Journal of Medicine*. Retrieved from www.nejm.org, e. 7(1–3)

Ruth. Link. Personal Approaches to Primary Care. Well Blog. New York Times .com. Retrieved from http://well.blogs.nytimes.com/2010/07/15/a-personal-approach-to-primary-care/

Sack, K. (2010, March 16). With Medicaid cuts, doctors and patients drop out. *The New York Times*, p. A1.

Scal, P. (2002). Transition for youth with chronic conditions: Primary care physicians' approaches. *Pediatrics*, 110, 1315–1321.

Schilling, B. (2009). *What is the patient-centered medical home?* The Commonwealth Fund. Retrieved from www.commonwealthfund.org/Content/Newsletters/

Schneider, E. (2010). *Chronic Disease Self-Management Program (CDSMP). Evidence-based chronic disease self-management program for older adults*. Chapel Hill, NC: University of North Carolina.

Schoen, C., Osborn, R., Squires, D., Doty, M. M., Pierson, R., and Applebaum, S. (2010, November 18). How health insurance design affects access to care and costs by income, in eleven countries. *In the literature, highlights from Commonwealth Fund-Supported Studies in Professional Journals*, pp. 1–2. New York City.

Schoenborn, C. A., and Heyman, K. M. (2009). Health characteristics of adults aged 55 years and over. United States. 2004–2007. National Health Statistics Reports: no. 16. Hyattsville, MD: National Center for Health Statistics.

Schram, A. P. (2010). Medical home and the nurse practitioner: A policy analysis. *Journal for Nurse Practitioners*, 6, 132–139.

Sebelius, K. (2010a). Medicare and the new health care law—what it means for you. Center for Medicare and Medicaid Services, Washington, DC, CMS Product No. 11467.

Sebelius, K. (2010b, July 26). Unpublished letter from the Secretary of Health and Human Services to the state governors on the anniversary of the Americans with Disabilities Act. Washington, DC: Department of Health and Human Services.

Seifter, J., with Seifter, B. (2010). *After the diagnosis: Transcending chronic illness.* New York: Simon and Shuster.

Seligman, H. K., and Schillinger, D. (2010). Hunger and socioeconomic disparities in chronic disease. *New England Journal of Medicine*, 363, 6–9.

Sen, A. (2010). *The idea of justice.* Cambridge, MA: Belknap Press/Harvard University Press.

Shannon, T. (2009, October, 28). *Transition care: A coordinated approach to discharge planning.* Presented at the New York State Health Care Foundation Conference, New York City.

Shipman, W. (2010). Link. Personal Approaches to Primary Care. Well Blog. New York Times.com. Retrieved from http://well.blogs.nytimes.com/2010/07/15/a-personal-approach-to-primary-care/

Shortell, S. M., Casalino, L. P., and Fisher, E. S. (2010). How the Center for Medicare and Medicaid Innovation should test accountable care organizations. *Health Affairs*, 29, 1293–1298.

Sidorov, J. E. (2008). The patient-centered medical home for chronic illness: Is it ready for prime time? *Health Affairs* 27, 1231–1234.

Simmons, A. M. (2010, October 29). Sick Californians may be forgoing care because health deductible is too high, study says. Retrieved from www.latimes.com/news/la-sickinsured28-m

Solomon, J. (2010). Health reform expands Medicaid coverage for people with disabilities. *Moving forward with health reform.* Washington, DC: Center for Budget and Policy Priorities, pp. 1–2.

Sontag, S. (1978, January 26). Illness as metaphor. *New York Review of Books*, 10–16.

Stanford University School of Medicine. (2010). Chronic disease self-management program. Retrieved from http://patienteducation.stanford.edu/programs/cdsmp.html

Stange, K. C., Nutting, P. A., Miller, W. L., Jaen, C. R., Crabtree, B. F., Flocke, S. A., and Gill, J. M. (2010). Defining and measuring the patient-centered medical home. *Journal of General Internal Medicine*, 25, 601–612.

Starfield, B., Lemke, K. W., Bernhardt, T., Foldess, S. S., Forrest, C. B., and Weiner, J. P. (2003). Comorbidity: Implications for the importance of primary care in "care management." *Annals of Family Medicine* (May/June), 1, 8–14.

Starfield, B., Shi, L., Macinko, J., Wagner, E. H., Austin, B. T., Davis, C., Hindmarsh, M., Schaefer, J., and Bonomi, A. (2001). Improving chronic illness care: Translating evidence into action. *Health Affairs*, 20, 64–78.

Steele, G. D., Haynes, J. A., Davis, D. E., Tomcavage, J., Stewart, W. F., Graf, T. R., Paulus, R. A., Weikel, K., and Shikles, J. (2010). How Geisinger's advanced medical home model argues the case for rapid-cycle innovation. *Health Affairs*, 29, 2047–2053.

Steinbrook, R. (2008). Health care reform in Massachusetts—expanding coverage, escalating costs. *New England Journal of Medicine*, 358, 2757–2760.

Stock, S., Drabik, A., Buscher, G., Graf, C., Ullrich, W., Gerber, A., Lauterbach, K. W. and Lungen, M. (2010). German diabetes management programs improve quality of care and curb costs. *Health Affairs*, 29, 2197–2205.

Stringhini, S., Sabia, S., Shipley, M., Brunner, E., Nabi, H., Kvimaki, M., and Singh-Manoux, A. (2010, March 24/31). Association of socioeconomic position with health behaviors and mortality. *Journal of the American Medical Association*, 303, 1159–1166.

Takach, M., Gauthier, A., Sims-Kastelein, K. and Kaye, N. (2010, December). Strengthening primary care: State innovations to transform and link small practices. New York City. National Academy for State Health Policy and the Commonwealth Fund, Publication no. 1459.

Thorpe, K. E. (2009, May 14). Statement of Kenneth E. Thorpe, Ph.D., at the Senate Committee on Health, Education, Labor and Pensions Hearing On: Delivery reform: The roles of primary and specialty care in innovative new delivery models. Dirksen 430, Washington, DC.

Thorpe, K. E., and Howard, D. A. (2006). The rise in spending among Medicare beneficiaries: The role of chronic disease prevalence and changes in treatment intensity. *Health Affairs, 25.* Web Exclusive, w378–388.

Thorpe, K., and Ogden, L. (2009, October 5). Creating the virtual integrated delivery system. *Health Affairs.* Retrieved from www.healthaffairs.org/ blog/20

Thorpe, K. E., Ogden, L. L., and Galactionova, K. (2010). Chronic conditions account for rise in Medicare spending from 1987 to 2006. *Health Affairs*, 29, 718–724.

Trivedi, A. N., Moloo, H., and Mor, V. (2010). Increased ambulatory care copayments and hospitalizations among the elderly. *New England Journal of Medicine* 362, 320–328.

United Hospital Fund. (2010). Cost sharing in New York's health insurance market. New York: United Hospital Fund.

U.S. Department of Health and Human Services. (2010). HHS announces the nation's new health promotion and disease prevention agenda. Washington, DC: OASH Press Office.

U.S. Department of Health and Human Services. Health Resources and Services Administration, Maternal and Child Health Bureau. (2008). *The National Survey of Children with Special Health Care Needs Chartbook 2005–2006.* Rockville, MD: Author.

Van Cleave, J., Gortmaker, S. L., and Perrin, J. M. (2010). Dynamics of obesity and chronic health conditions among children and youth. *Journal of the American Medical Association*, 303, 623–630.

Varney, S. (2010, January 4). Congress proposes new physician payment system. National Public Radio, San Francisco, CA, KQED.

Voelker, R. (2008). US health care system earns poor marks. *Journal of the American Medical Association*, 300, 2843–2844.

Weinstein, M. C., and Skinner, J. A. (2010). Comparative effectiveness and health care spending—implications for reform. *New England Journal of Medicine*, 362, 460–465.

White, P. H. (2009). Destination known: Planning the transition of youth with special health care needs to adult health care. *Adolescent Health Update*, 21, 1–8.

Whittle, P. (2009, July 29). Wheelchair worries: Bethpage firm's move to halt sales leaves disabled LIers in limbo. *Newsday,* p. A13.

Wikipedia, thc free encyclopedia. (2009). Medical home. Retrieved from http://en.wikipedia.org/wiki/Medical-home

Wilensky, G. R. (2009). The policies and politics of creating a comparative clinical effectiveness research center. *Health Affairs.* 28, w719–w729. Web exclusive. Retrieved from 10.1377/hlthaff.28.4w719

Xu, J., Kochanek K. D., and Tejada-Vera, B. (2009). Preliminary data for 2007. National Vital Statistics Reports; 58. Hyattesville, MD: National Center for Health Statistics.

Zuckerman, S., Merrell, K., Berenson, R., Gans, D. N., Underwood, W. S., Williams, A., Erickson, S. M., and Hammons, T. (2009, October). *Incremental cost estimates for the patient-centered medical home.* New York: The Commonwealth Fund.

Zuger, A. (2008, February 28). For the very old, a dose of "slow medicine." *New York Times,* p. D6.

# Index

About the Author

ARNOLD BIRENBAUM is a Professor of Pediatrics at the Albert Einstein College of Medicine and Associate Director of the Rose F. Kennedy University Center for Excellence in Developmental Disability Education, Research and Service. His background and interests are in medical sociology and health policy analysis, which he employs in attempting to improve the U.S. health care system. Degreed in sociology at Columbia University, he has also been a Professor of Sociology at St. John's University and an Assistant Professor of Sociology at City College of New York and an Associate Professor of Sociology at Wheaton College.